BREATHTAKING

Breathtaking

ASTHMA CARE IN A TIME OF CLIMATE CHANGE

Alison Kenner

University of Minnesota Press
Minneapolis
London

Published by the University of Minnesota Press
111 Third Avenue South, Suite 290
Minneapolis, MN 55401–2520
http://www.upress.umn.edu

Printed in the United States of America on acid-free paper

The University of Minnesota is an equal-opportunity educator and employer.

24 23 22 21 20 19 18   10 9 8 7 6 5 4 3 2 1

Library of Congress Cataloging-in-Publication Data
Names: Kenner, Alison, author.
Title: Breathtaking : asthma care in a time of climate change / Alison Kenner.
Description: Minneapolis : University of Minnesota Press, [2018] | Includes bibliographical references and index. |
Identifiers: LCCN 2018008958 (print) | ISBN 978-1-5179-0286-5 (hc) | ISBN 978-1-5179-0287-2 (pb)
Subjects: | MESH: Asthma–therapy. | Asthma–etiology. | Breathing Exercises. | Respiratory Physiological Phenomena. | Climate Change.
Classification: LCC RC591 (print) | NLM WF 553 | DDC 616.2/38–dc23
LC record available at https://lccn.loc.gov/2018008958

To all those with asthma,
and those who care for asthma,
who helped me understand what it means
to live in an unbreathable world

CONTENTS

Introduction   1

1 Attuning to Asthma in Time and Place   29

2 Three Modes of Control as Asthma Care   57

3 Counting on Breath:
   Making Time with Respiratory Retraining   85

4 The Datafication of Care   115

5 Public Health Carescapes for Climate Change   149

   Conclusion   177

   Acknowledgments   187

   Notes   191

   Bibliography   209

   Index   225

I wake up to his breathing.

I roll over to find him seated, hunched over the edge of the bed. I say nothing but am immediately alert; this is the kind of thing that wakes you up out of a dead sleep. I lie there, a foot away, watching and listening. I wonder if he will tell me if he needs to go to the hospital, or if he will try to leave me out of his asthma attack altogether. I know from previous experience not to reach out to him. I don't know what suffocation feels like, but for Jess, touch is not a welcome gesture when he's struggling to breathe. He needs space and silence. These things are opposite to how I responded the first and second time asthma struck in the night. The first time it happened I touched his back and asked questions. Now I know to just listen: to air scraping against his narrowed trachea, the audible wheeze; to the controlled pacing of inhale and exhale, intuitively measured by his sense of lung capacity; to the momentary stillness of the pause he takes at both ends of each breath.

I close my eyes again. Jess will stay in his hunched position until the wheeze goes away. It could be a half hour or forty-five minutes, maybe longer. I open my eyes. You need to be ready, I tell myself. Don't get comfortable. Although this space, the space of asthma, has become familiar to me through my research and personal life, asthma cannot be taken for granted. It is a wily thing that can turn deadly. Care in the moment of an asthma attack needs to be disciplined, rhythmic, and controlled—the mode that Jess enacts on the edge of the bed, with his breathing body. But care also needs to be attuned and responsive. So I listen with sharp attention.

Readers familiar with asthma may note what I have not mentioned in the above picture: a rescue inhaler. Salbutamol, more commonly known as albuterol, is a bronchodilator that relaxes airway muscles. Delivered through an inhaler, it is used at the onset of asthma symptoms: wheezing, chest tightness, breathlessness, coughing. The albuterol rescue inhaler is the most common medication prescribed and used for asthma. On this night Jess doesn't have a rescue inhaler. Although he has lived with asthma for more than twenty-five years, it's been more than a decade since he's had health insurance.[1] He hasn't seen a doctor for asthma in more than five years, not since the time he went to urgent care for a really bad attack. He had no inhaler then either. In lieu of medical care from a doctor, Jess receives hand-me-down rescue inhalers from his father. He uses these only when absolutely necessary. Otherwise, he just deals with low-grade disordered breathing using ad hoc strategies and embodied techniques—controlling his breath, drinking coffee, sometimes leaving a space that is triggering symptoms.

Jess's father, Randy, has allergic asthma too, but he doesn't need the rescue inhaler he has been prescribed. Randy uses an inhaler with a controller medication each morning to prevent asthma symptoms altogether. Controller medications are prescribed for people who suffer from allergic asthma or more severe forms of the disease. Randy refills two prescriptions each month, both the controller and rescue inhalers, even though he doesn't need the latter. He gives his rescue inhalers to Jess, so his son will always have one. Tonight, however, there is nothing in the house to open Jess's airways; his father's rescue inhaler has been missing for more than a week. But Jess isn't panicked: nighttime attacks are familiar if terrifying terrain for him. His self-designed breathing ritual is based on years of experience with asthma in all kinds of situations. His strategy—sitting on the edge of the bed, pacing his breath with intense but calm focus—is not just about bringing his breath back to a state of normal. It's a tactic for staying calm in the face of suffocation. To combat the attack and bring his breath back to normal, Jess needs to relax as best he can.

Still lying on my side, listening to the rhythm of his breath, I assign the pace and depth of his breath meaning, hoping that it will give me a sense of his state. I try to assess how each breath sounds against the last, and the ones to come, and how these strained movements measure against others from similar after-midnight asthma attacks I have listened to. I imagine Jess doing a similar but different assessment, drawing on a sensory register embedded in his lungs and throat and nerves—a sensory register that I don't have access to. I make my own assessment, listening to the flow and texture of his breath. It helps to close the gap between us, an arm's length that feels like a mile in this moment.

As I listen to the rhythm of air against his body, I run through a list of things that could have triggered Jess's attack. Without a rescue inhaler,

Jess had been much more thoughtful, careful, than usual about where he went and what he did this last week. He told his boss at the construction company where he works that he would not be able to do demolition or painting until he got a new inhaler—a request that his boss respected. On a job site, in an unfamiliar place, with people around, it would be much harder to control an asthma attack. It's risky enough for someone with asthma to enter an unfamiliar building. When doctors prescribe asthma medications, indoor environments are one of the first things they ask patients about. Old homes often breed mold and harbor pests, and owners and tenants use all kinds of chemicals and pesticides to keep these asthma triggers in check. Jess spends time in exactly these kinds of places in his work renovating old Philadelphia row houses. And predictably, he feels that indoor environments are the most problematic for him. But there are larger, atmospheric and ecological, dynamics at play as well, which I like to remind him of, even if I have failed to convince him of their significance.

Time of year is important for asthma and its care, too. On this night, it's the last weekend in October, and Jess has always said that dry leaves trigger his symptoms, that his asthma is at its worst in the fall. Indoor heating systems are coming on for the first time in six or seven months, kicking dust out into domestic breathing spaces. I also think about the archived study I read a month ago, which found that Philadelphia children experience more asthma symptoms in the fall because of weather patterns and air pollution.[2] Compared with other cities in the United States, Philadelphia has higher asthma prevalence rates, worse morbidity from asthma, and poorer health care outcomes for those with asthma.[3] When I talk to Philadelphians about their health, many tell me they suspect that city air pollution contributes to their breathing problems.

Work exposure, dilapidated housing stock, and city air quality aside, we had spent the weekend moving me into Jess's apartment. This stirred up materials of all kinds, including dust and residue from a mixture of cleaning products. Things from my old place that would not have been in Jess's space previously, including a feather down pillow, throw rugs, and dander from my roommate's cat, were now affecting the air quality. Jess is a meticulous cleaner—yet another strategy he uses to manage his asthma—and undoubtedly my stuff has thrown off his indoor environment. The structures of asthma science coupled with clinical discourse make it easy to frame these experiences as the fault of domestic doings and individualized moves. But I remind myself that it is not any one of these exposures or contexts that has created this moment of narrowed airways and audible breath. Jess's asthma attack is the result of structural conditions produced by material-cultural densities that have come together, accumulating and building on past exposures and conditions, to create a particular event in a world that more and more people are finding increasingly unbreathable.[4]

Twenty-five minutes later, the pace of Jess's breathing has slowed to what I would call normal. It's less punctuated by the suspensions he employs at the top and bottom of each breath. Jess stands up and grabs an empty glass from the nightstand. I listen to water from the faucet filling the glass, and half a minute later the TV comes on. I know he doesn't want to lie back down, flattening his now rejuvenated lungs between gravity and the mattress.

Jess's story presents a very common, age-old manifestation of asthma, in which the breather wakes in the middle of the night breathless, coughing, in the midst of an asthma attack.[5] It is a scene depicted across the asthma literature and described in scores of the interviews I conducted for this book. But another form of asthma has also helped shape this book's narrative and argument, a form of asthma that is collective, public, and may become more common.

I learned of thunderstorm asthma from an article describing a forty-eight-hour epidemic that struck London in the summer of 1994. During the event, more than 2,000 residents from southeast England, including London and its suburbs, sought medical care for asthma symptoms. More than 1,500 people made do with general care practitioners and on-call physicians, but 640 Londoners fled to a dozen emergency rooms. Many of those who sought emergency care were already living with an asthma diagnosis, but 44 percent (283 people) had never before experienced breathing difficulty. Hospitals were unprepared for the magnitude of this event. Many ran out of the necessary supplies: medications, nebulizers, and even mouthpieces for peak flow meters. Extra doctors had to be called in from other locations. The epidemic caught the entire region off guard.[6]

The cause or, better yet, "trigger" of the London asthma epidemic was a severe thunderstorm. As the storm traveled to the northeast across London, the temperature dropped and the wind picked up, creating a powerful vertical air current. Next came rain and a rapid increase in humidity. These weather patterns produced a dramatic rise in the aeroallergen count, a measure of airborne materials capable of producing allergic reactions when inhaled. When the storm arrived, the city's air pollution levels were already elevated: grass pollen counts were the highest they had been in six years, and the concentration of particulate matter on the day of the storm was the highest it had been all year. In other words, an intense meteorological event (the storm) collided with a particularly ripe surface atmosphere (pollution).[7]

Of course, only those most severely affected by the storm would have visited emergency departments. The tenfold increase in patient visits at London hospitals for asthma after the storm misses those who might have managed symptoms at home—perhaps those who were less severely affected by the storm, or people already diagnosed with asthma who recognized the attacks and had rescue inhalers on hand. Some, too, may have been protected by daily pharmaceutical regimens designed to prevent symptoms in any environment, all the time. This latter group could in some ways be considered proof that daily medication for asthma control works as it should. But a person's location in relation to atmospheric events matters too. In a study conducted in Atlanta, Georgia, researchers found that a high percentage of those affected by thunderstorm asthma were outdoors when the thunderstorm hit.[8]

Scientists predict that such flash asthma epidemics will become more frequent as climate change progresses, as extreme weather events become more common, pollen counts rise, and allergy seasons start earlier and last longer.[9] Climate change is influencing the way asthma is experienced and the types of responses that are needed. The growing number of people with seasonal allergies and asthma means that more people will be affected by extreme weather events. Twenty years after the London incident and on the other side of the world, an even more devastating thunderstorm asthma event hit Melbourne, Australia, killing nine people and sending more than ten thousand to emergency medical care facilities for asthma treatment.[10] Now more than ever we need to care for the place of breathing in the world.

Together, the two scenes described above index the intimate and public valences of asthma. Both also cast asthma as an event, a moment of "attack," a depiction that has come to stand in for the disease in cultural imaginaries. While asthma attacks highlight the life-threatening potential of disordered breathing—the side of asthma we know from the news, public health campaigns, experiences with friends and family members, and possibly our own lives—these events also render invisible the accumulations, the chronicity, the mundane, low-grade, normalized dynamics of environmental health.[11] The daily care practices that guard against asthma attacks are also rendered invisible by the focus on events. In this book, I attempt to hold various timescapes of breathing and its disorder together—its histories, events, and futures—by documenting the ways in which care is enacted across different scales and places, from the intimate moments of listening to the breath to health literacy campaigns that communicate the impacts of climate change.

I use the term *breathers*—borrowed from cultural anthropologist Tim Choy—to point to the breadth and multiplicity of breathing contexts and affects described in this book. Choy explains that environmental economists use the term to document how people accrue the unaccounted-for costs of industrial and economic activities. It is also a "vacuous" term, Choy observes: Who is not a breather?[12] How does this term allow us to account for the costs of late industrialism, environmental degradation, and climate change? Asthma is one form of these costs, a cost that has shown up across populations, measured in prevalence and hospitalization rates, mortality, and prescription medication use. But even *asthma* has been a contested term and one limited in its reach, for reasons that I will explore in chapter 1.[13]

Symptoms resembling asthma have been described in medical and literary texts for more than two thousands years, yet today's changing ecologies, health care systems, medical sciences, and built environments are reshaping the disease.[14] Now identified as a global epidemic, asthma—along with efforts to control it and its intricate relationship to changing environments—demands an analysis that is attentive to the disease's complexity and its contextual nature, as well as the care practices that emerge from both. The chapters that follow join a rich historical literature with a contemporary perspective provided by interviews with people who live with asthma today. They also extend the existing asthma literature by situating illness experiences in relation to environmental rhythms and qualities, biopolitical economies, chemical and digital technologies, and emplaced modes of knowing. Empirically and analytically, the arguments that I make in this book are based on cases that highlight the different scales and spaces through which asthma is produced and addressed—markets, seasons, storms, social events, movements, and relationships between humans and nonhumans. The case of asthma and its care also offers new insight into the relationships among environment, time, and human health more broadly—a topic of particular salience today.

In this book I advance three arguments about asthma care in the United States. The first argument builds on the assertion that care practices are context-specific.[15] They are attuned to the environment and structured through time in deeply embodied ways. Asthma sufferers feel the air as heavy or textured. They detect smells that signal the presence of smoke or mold. They (or their caregivers) detect, or sometimes fail to detect, signs in the body that indicate that contact has been made with chemicals or allergens such as animal dander or tree pollen. People with asthma are also affected by and attuned to their movements within and between places. This can be as simple as attuning to the transition between outdoor and indoor environments, seasonal changes, or differences in air quality between geographic regions. People with asthma also take pollution and other environmental factors into consideration when planning residential moves or when traveling. Sensory knowledge, which is built from embodied memory and meaning making, is a core component of care for asthma sufferers.[16]

Asthma care is also enacted at various temporal scales, which may be expressed as care time or care rhythms.[17] These scales include the respiratory rhythms Jess used in breathing through his nighttime asthma attack. Care time also includes the day-to-day timing of medication regimens and seasonal variations in disordered breathing, which are entangled with changes in such environmental factors as temperature, pollen count, industrial pollution, and viral transmission. For some asthmatics, cold and flu season is the most detrimental time of the year, because getting sick activates their asthma. Changes over the life course also affect how asthma is experienced and cared for. My emphasis on time and place thus reflects how those I interviewed talked about the emplaced and temporally situated dynamics of asthma, as well as the way asthma is framed as an environmental health issue in communities, in cities, and at the national scale.

My second argument relates to pharmaceutical treatments as a relatively recent innovation in asthma management, one situated in the era of biomedicalization. Medical sociologists use the term *biomedicalization* to refer to the technoscientific transformations that have changed the practice, organization, and constitution of biomedicine since the mid-1980s. Although prescription medications for asthma have been available for more than half a century, today's recommended pharmaceutical regimens, as well as those under development, exemplify many elements of biomedicalization, including technoscientific identities that are shaped by the rhythms of medication use and pulmonary assessments, regimens of surveillance and control oriented toward future risk and health, and clinical research that aims to identify and classify asthma "types" at smaller and smaller scales of biological difference.[18] By situating pharmaceutical recommendations and care regimens for asthma in the era of biomedicalization, I signal the increased emphasis on the technoscientific elements that shape disease management discourse and infrastructure, making certain modes of care possible.

Understanding how asthma sufferers use (or do not use) prescription drugs requires not only an awareness of biomedicalization but also close attention to the environmental dimensions of disordered breathing and the structural conditions that make pharmaceutical treatments possible. Asthmatics use medications in a range of ways, sometimes following prescribed treatments to the letter and sometimes improvising according to social, environmental, or economic circumstances. Some asthma sufferers resist medication use, sometimes out of fear that their ability to breathe will become drug dependent. In other cases, medications fail to provide relief from symptoms, leaving asthmatics to search for and experiment with other modes of care. Tracing the context, value, and failures of pharmaceutical treatments can lead to important insights into both the disease and its care.

My final argument concerns how, in the U.S. context, contemporary approaches to environmental health have largely emphasized individual responsibility over collective responsibility. While some modes of care described here mirror practices that have been written about through asthma's history, other responses—both public and private—reflect unique circumstances of the contemporary epidemic as well as advances in biomedicine and pharmaceutical treatments. I join with other social science researchers in arguing that asthma care has been individualized in neoliberal ways; even public health responses have tended to emphasize the responsibility of individuals—taking medication, cleaning home environments, and monitoring pulmonary performance—over collective responsibility.[19] Recent attempts to enact stronger environmental policy, particularly in the United States, have fallen devastatingly short of what is needed to protect respiratory health. The modes of care profiled in this book expose the tensions and relationships between individualizing responses and collective frameworks that govern environmental health issues.[20] Yet I also show how care is always embedded in broader systems and relations of care—care infrastructures, carescapes, webs of care, nested dependencies, and human–nonhuman relations.[21] Toward the end of the book, I show how new modes of collective care practices may be generating a kind of public health that can address the asthma epidemic in this time of climate change.

A Contemporary Epidemic

In the modern era, asthma is one of several disease conditions that may be diagnosed when an individual has reoccurring breathing difficulty. Asthma can be experienced as wheezing, coughing, chest tightness, shortness of breath, or, in extreme cases, a complete inability to breathe. These symptoms can be experienced in mild or severe form, persistently or as acute events. Asthma symptoms may be triggered by exposure to ground ozone, tobacco smoke, cold air, chemicals and odors, pet dander, pollen, viruses, and stress, among other things.[22] Environmental exposures like these may *cause* asthma, too—but that is up for evidence-based debate. Also included in recent theories of causation is exposure to viruses, pesticides, cockroaches, and polycyclic aromatic hydrocarbons, along with the absence of exposure to Vitamin D and protective bacteria (sometimes referred to as the hygiene hypothesis).[23]

Asthma is a complex disease condition that looks different from one person to the next. Symptoms and triggers differ from person to person, as do disease severity and responses to medications. Age of onset varies as well, and for those who live with asthma across the life course, the disease can change over time, taking on new forms. Asthma's variable and multiple quality may be compounded by a change of residence or relocation to a completely new ecology where the individual is exposed to seasonal cycles, climates, pollution sources and dynamics, pollen and humidity, and building conditions that are different from those experienced previously.

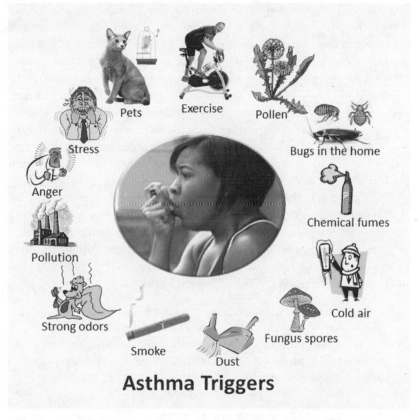

Asthma Triggers

During the period when this study was conducted, this image was the most common result of a Google search for "asthma triggers." Many versions of this figure exist; this one was the most frequently found at the time. Image by 7mike5000; courtesy of Wikimedia Commons.

Many people develop asthma before the age of eighteen, either during childhood or in their teenage years, and much research has been focused on this population group. Studies of occupational asthma have also contributed understanding to medical accounts of disordered breathing and its development. In recent years, medical researchers have paid increasing attention to adult-onset asthma, which may be related to phenotypes, endotypes, and exposure pathways that are not well understood.[24]

There is no cure for asthma. The disease is managed with several kinds of medications, behavioral interventions, and environmental control practices. Rescue inhalers, for example, are used almost universally by those diagnosed with asthma to combat symptoms as they emerge. For those with more than mild or intermittent asthma, a daily medication may be prescribed to prevent symptoms by controlling ongoing airway inflammation. In cases where asthma accompanies allergies, allergy shots and other medications may also be used. Many asthma sufferers adjust their behaviors and lifestyles, too, and attempt to avoid triggers and control their environments by modifying their homes. These are age-old, foundational modes of care, clinically recommended in the contemporary context alongside pharmaceutical treatments. These disease dynamics—the chronic and episodic states of asthma, its embeddedness in time and place, and the way the disease varies from patient to patient—demand a multifaceted analysis of the care practices enacted to address asthma in individuals and populations.

Tension between the lived experiences of disordered breathing, particularly across the life course, and modern medicine can be seen in a statement by a leading international asthma researcher, Dr. Fernando Martinez, a pediatrician who has served on the U.S. Food and Drug Administration's Pulmonary-Allergy Drugs Advisory Committee and the National Institutes of Health's expert panel for asthma management:

> Asthma is heterogeneous, and there are many different forms of the disease. In fact, sometimes I tell audiences that, you know, until very late in the nineteenth century fever was considered a disease. The same probably will be said about asthma twenty or thirty or fifty years from now. . . . Those of us who treat asthma know that it's very different in each person. It's almost as if each person is an *n* of one.[25]

This statement, quoted in an editorial in the medical journal *The Lancet*, has been joined by declarations that the term *asthma* is outdated and should be abandoned altogether.[26] Often these recommendations are coupled with observations about the complexity and heterogeneity of asthma as a disease. Gary P. Anderson, in discussing the reigning immunological model of asthma in a 2008 review, has noted that the model "cannot account for the substantial clinical and molecular heterogeneity that has now been unequivocally documented in human asthma. . . . This intellectual framework needs to revised. Indeed, that the entry criteria for patients into almost all clinical trials for asthma does not reflect the pattern of actual asthma in the community is remarkable."[27]

The intellectual framework that Anderson refers to is the Th2-inflammation hypothesis, which assumes that asthma is principally an immunological disease. The problem is that more and more people without the Th2-inflammation component are being diagnosed with asthma. If asthma is more than an allergic disease, what kind of disease is it? Is it, as Martinez suggests, a spectrum of diseases that present as disordered breathing? This question cannot be answered if clinical studies into the condition do not better represent the disease's heterogeneous spectrum, as Anderson suggests.

A different terminological problem exists among individuals diagnosed with asthma. Over time, as their illnesses and, by extension, their care practices change, many people question whether an asthma diagnosis actually applies to them. As I show in chapter 1, people often believe they have "grown out of" asthma because their experience of disordered breathing is no longer as severe and routine as it was during childhood. They may continue to experience breathlessness, allergies, wheezing, and other symptoms of asthma, but under different conditions. People in those circumstances often interpret disordered breathing as just latent effects of a childhood illness that they no longer have. The episodic and transformative dimensions of asthma—both of which stem from the emplaced condition of the disease—have led epidemiologists to develop three distinct questions for use in tracking national prevalence rates. The first concerns the presence of asthma over the individual's lifetime: Has the person ever received an asthma diagnosis? The second question addresses the person's current asthma status: Has the individual received an asthma diagnosis and has he or she been treated for asthma in the past twelve months? The final question concerns the prevalence of asthma attacks: How many asthma attacks has the individual had in the past twelve months? According to the CDC's National Health Survey, for example, almost 50 percent of people with current asthma had one or more asthma attacks in 2015.[28] This final question is used to assess the proportion of asthma sufferers whose conditions may be untreated or undertreated.[29] The temporality of this question set suggests that certain aspects of asthma's most commonly understood identity—an inability to breathe—may be rendered illegible as the disease changes over time and place.[30]

When asthma prevalence rates jumped in the United States in the 1980s, some commentators asked whether an expanded diagnostic framework could explain the apparent rise in disordered breathing. Some suspected that pharmaceutical development and new marketing tactics were affecting clinical practice. Such factors, however, could not explain the increases in asthma mortality and hospitalization rates that paralleled the rising national prevalence rates.[31] While some epidemiologists have suggested that other respiratory conditions, particularly those found in infants, older adults, and athletes, may have increasingly been diagnosed as asthma over the years, on the whole, new clinical practices alone could not explain the rise in prevalence rates.[32] According to the Centers for Disease Control and Prevention, from 2001 to 2010 the number of U.S. residents with asthma increased from 20.3 million to 25.7 million, an increase of almost 3 percent each year. During the same period, current asthma prevalence rates increased 1.5 percent per year, which meant that more people were experiencing and treating their asthma. At the same time, asthma attack prevalence decreased slightly.[33] Some research has suggested that the decrease in asthma attacks alongside higher rates of asthma means that more people are taking medications (and responding yes when asked about current asthma) but are having fewer attacks. Asthma management regimens are working as they should, in other words. While federal epidemiological data have shown that lifetime prevalence rates have begun to plateau— findings that mirror trends in other countries with similar asthma profiles— other asthma researchers point out that federal data collection methods are limited and likely miss the most vulnerable population groups: adults and children living in poverty, those living in rural areas (with limited access to medical care), and those experiencing homelessness.[34]

The U.S. asthma epidemic has had its greatest impacts on children and on African Americans. The CDC has reported that national prevalence rates increased by 75 percent between 1980 and 1996, with disproportionate increases in both these groups. The disparities have persisted over time.[35] The proportion of children who had experienced asthma in the past twelve months more than doubled from 1980 to 1995, from 3.6 percent to 7.5 percent. Prevalence in children under the age of five increased 160 percent during this period. From 2001 to 2010, the rate of childhood asthma prevalence increase slowed, but it still rose from 8.7 percent to 9.3 percent over the decade. Until recently, asthma rates among children showed little variation across race, but new studies show racial disparities emerging among asthma sufferers under the age of eighteen.[36]

Among adults, disparities between African Americans and whites in asthma prevalence rates have been an ongoing trend. Between 2001 and 2010, asthma prevalence among both Hispanic and black populations increased at a rate of 3.2 percent a year, more than twice the increase (1.4 percent) in white persons.[37] Prevalence rates from more recent years have continued these trends. Racial disparities in adverse disease outcomes, including hospitalizations and death, have been tracked in all age groups since the 1980s and have held steady over the decades. Adult women have also been disproportionately affected by asthma, with higher prevalence rates, higher mortality, and worse treatment outcomes than adult men.

These jumps in asthma prevalence rates, as well as the race, gender, and age disparities, have propelled new research on disease causation. Large and well-funded research programs have focused on genetic and molecular pathways, including prenatal exposure and biological susceptibility.[38] Many researchers hope that these studies will lend insight into disease mechanisms that will allow for the development of targeted treatments. To date, however, population-based research on biological differences has not produced results, reflecting the very broad terrain of factors connected to asthma. Indeed, many other researchers have criticized the focus on biological difference, pointing out that poverty and low socioeconomic status are greater risk factors than race, gender, age, and location alone in prevalence and treatment outcomes.[39]

While asthma scientists continue to work to understand the biochemical mechanisms of the disease in order to develop more effective treatments, the costs of currently available asthma drugs have increased dramatically in recent years. A searing 2013 *New York Times* article headlined "The Soaring Cost of a Simple Breath" reported that the price of an albuterol inhaler, the rescue inhaler that has saved lives for decades, had increased from $15 to $50 or even $100 (in some places) in recent years.[40] In 2014, a congressional report showed that the market price of one hundred albuterol tablets (2 mg) had jumped from $11 in October 2013 to $434 in April 2014, an increase of 4,014 percent.[41] Although albuterol had been off-patent for decades, the drug was repatented when a ban on chlorofluorocarbons (CFCs) in 2005 called for a new inhaler design. An oft-cited justification for the high cost of asthma medications is that the systems used to deliver them are protected by layers of patents. The CFC ban and associated product design update led to "large relative increases in out-of-pocket albuterol costs among privately insured individuals with asthma and modest declines in utilization," according to one study; "the policy's impact on individuals without insurance, who faced greater cost increases, is unknown."[42] There are no generic inhalers, and few cost breaks are

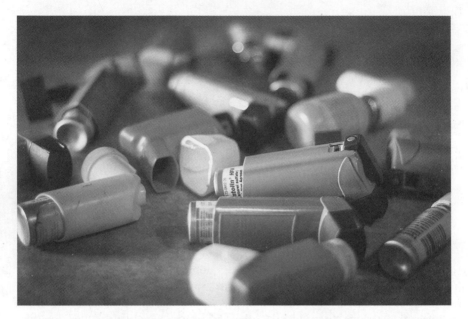

Most of the breathers I interviewed described using rescue inhalers. Some talked about how quickly they use up their rescue inhalers, depending on the time of year, for example. A few mentioned that they had bedroom or kitchen drawers filled with empty inhaler canisters. Photograph by Jack Lawrence; courtesy of Flickr.

available, even through federal and state health programs. California's Medicaid program, for example, spent $61 million in 2012 for asthma drugs, often paying more than $200 per inhaler.[43]

Rescue inhalers are just one of many types of medications used to manage asthma; many people with asthma are prescribed several kinds of drugs. Controller medications are used to prevent attacks; one expensive example is a combination inhaler that contains a bronchodilator and a corticosteroid. Allergy medicines are also often prescribed for people with asthma. Given the high price of inhalers (and the other kinds of drugs prescribed to manage the disease), many people report that they try to minimize drug use for financial reasons. "I minimize puffs to minimize costs," a woman told *New York Times* reporters. Even with good health insurance, patients can easily pay more than $1,000 each year for these medications.[44] Many of the people I interviewed reported that it seemed like the prices changed every time they went to the pharmacy.

Lack of access to health care and affordable medicine is a leading factor in mortality and other adverse effects of asthma, such as poor quality of life and risk of falling into poverty.[45] In 2013, for example, asthma resulted in 1.6 million emergency department visits across the United States.[46] Although death from asthma is highly preventable, thousands die from the disease each year in the United States. According to CDC data, 3,615 people died from asthma in 2015, 59 percent of whom were women; 168 more people died from asthma in 2015 than in 2007.[47] Predictors of death include three or more emergency department visits in the past year, a hospitalization or emergency department visit in the past month, over-use of rescue medication, difficulty perceiving asthma symptoms, lack of an asthma action plan, low socioeconomic status, and being female, non-white, a smoker, or suffering from major mental health issues or other medical conditions, such as cardiovascular disease.

According to the CDC, asthma care costs the United States more than $81 billion each year. That figure includes the costs of medication, emergency department visits, hospitalizations, and missed school and work days.[48] Most reports focus on the costs of untreated asthma, which leads to emergency department use, missed school and work days, and hospitalizations. Few reports address the exorbitant costs of medications and the economic and structural barriers to accessing health care; such obstacles drive up the costs of asthma by placing preventive care out of reach for many people. Even fewer reports discuss how environmental regulations and resources to address exposures in the built environment might help reduce the national cost of asthma. All of these factors—the heterogeneity of the disease, the episodic dimension of the illness, the intersection of environmental and demographic factors, poverty, the exorbitant costs of medication, and inadequate national health care—can make asthma difficult to care for on many levels.

Five Iterations of Care

Through this project I have considered the varied ways in which asthma care is enacted: in the checking of daily weather reports and the use of medication; in breathing exercises, cleaning rituals, and avoidance measures; in the efforts of school nurses, coaches, parents, partners, friends, doctors, and community health workers who aid asthma sufferers in the moment of attack, as well as in daily rituals and periodic checkups; in the advocacy work of nonprofits and community organizations, which has led to state policies that allow students to carry inhalers in schools and to laws against vehicle idling in some cities; and in the epidemiological research of government agencies, the exposure studies conducted by interdisciplinary scientists, and the ontological debates engaged in by asthma experts. And, of course, technologies enact care, too.[49]

Care has long been an important analytic framework for describing relationships, particularly those related to illness, dependence, and governance. Care has been used as an ethical framework, a descriptive device, and an explanatory logic by feminist philosophers and social scientists, nurses and other health care professionals, anthropologists, and scholars in science and technology studies—disciplinary distinctions that are often blurred for those writing about care. As a framework for thinking through ethical-political positions, care has provided a window into relationships between caregiver and cared-for, and between governments and populations; it offers a way of thinking through human and nonhuman relations, as well as a way to situate researchers and their subjects in the context of knowledge production. Care enacts ethics through material practice in ways that reproduce and coproduce power, difference, and inequalities, which are always entrenched in social, economic, and cultural legacies.[50]

In this book, I explore asthma in its contemporary form by describing different modes of care for disordered breathing through individual responses, communities of practice, and programs that address the epidemic in the United States. Care in this context is focused on material practices and relations.[51] I describe five modes of care, using examples that reflect how asthma is addressed at different sociocultural scales; these modes are attuning, controlling, making care time, infrastructuring, and creating carescapes. Sometimes these modes of care work in combination, building from or preceding one another. Sometimes the connections are dynamic and impossible to parse. There are overlaps and also tensions between different modes of care. By documenting and comparing these five forms, I aim to show how care works across scales.[52] One reason to track asthma care across scales in this way is to show how care always exceeds the self. This is particularly important to highlight in the current era of biomedicalization, when an emphasis on the individual makes it easy to lose sight of the structures of power, economic dynamics, and technoscientific fields that shape possibilities for care. Tracing experiences of and responses to asthma in time and place provides a rich description of the variety of relationships and emplacements that produce care in different forms.

I use the concept of *asthmatic attunement* to describe the affective experiences that many asthma sufferers relayed to me in interviews. Asthmatic attunement involves the way in which a breather experiences the world through environmental qualities, specifically atmospheric conditions such as the thickness of air, its texture and scent, and temperature.[53] Asthmatic attunement often stems from sensations in the lungs and airways, including chest tightness, itchiness in the throat, a cough, and other signs of disordered breathing. Sometimes attunement to environmental conditions precedes asthma symptoms, particularly if the person has lived with disordered breathing for many years. Memories of how the atmosphere affects breathing enable the person to tune in to the present place, and to notice how the world feels on the body before a disordered response. Attunement is an embodied state that may be foundational for a breather's practice of asthma care. Like other modes of embodiment, attunement provides an orientation to the unbreathable world and shapes responses to it.[54]

Controlling is a very different mode of care. If attuning is anchored in sensing, controlling is a related mode of embodied care that tries to direct or restrain the situation that the body is attuning to. Controlling means exerting power over something. In the context of disease, it can be a means to reduce the impact or spread of illness, particularly when understood through a public health perspective. Control works through techniques or activities that employ power with varying degrees of force. Asthma sufferers, for example, engage in nuanced breath control techniques as they attune to emergent symptoms. These techniques respond to asthma by directing the breath in ways that help mediate symptoms and keep the breather calm in the face of an oncoming attack.

In this context, control is a mode of care. While other scholars have opposed the two—care and control—for a person with asthma, to be able to direct and restrict the breath when symptoms arise *is* care.[55] It is a response-in-the-now that leverages time and place through embodied engagement. The practice of breath control in response to asthma symptoms is part of many well-developed techniques and routines. Breathers may learn these techniques and routines from caregivers who help coach them through asthma attacks. Breath control tactics also involve an embodied tinkering with breath in the space of an attack, where the breather is "attending to the balances inside, and the flows between, a fragile body and its intricate surroundings."[56]

People with asthma also enact environmental control practices to reduce exposure to known or potential triggers. Such practices include avoidance strategies, regimented cleaning, and more extensive material interventions in home environments. This mode of care often stems from asthmatic attunement, which helps breathers identify what materials and situations trigger asthma. It is also a clinically recommended mode of care. Indeed, environmental control practices have long been a mainstay of asthma treatment.[57] Attention to this mode of controlled care also reveals much about how vulnerability is produced in place and time, shaped by a structural violence that prevents or makes it exponentially more difficult for some people to control their exposures. Environmental control practices, in other words, may be more necessary in some contexts than in others, and yet in the contexts where control may be most needed, these practices are the most difficult to implement.

The language of control came up repeatedly in my interviews with asthma sufferers, who used it to refer to how they care for disordered breathing, but control is also part of the discursive currency used to assess and treat asthma in the clinic. Control in the clinic is concerned with the management of disease indicators; this is quite different from the attuned and emplaced care practices that asthma sufferers describe in the language of control. In the clinic, a patient's asthma is assessed according to various dimensions of disordered breathing; successful disease management is referred to as *asthma control*. Asthma control is most often achieved with controller medications, which are taken daily to reduce airway inflammation. Controller medications keep symptoms at bay in the present, but they also protect asthma sufferers from the risk of future symptoms and irreversible damage to the airways.[58] In clinical contexts, asthma control is a measure of the success of patient care. In chapter 2, I explore how these different understandings and uses of the term *control* matter in asthma care arenas.

Both attuning and controlling are modes of care that rely on time and place; both practices involve making care time for asthma in different ways. Barbara Adam has used the term *timescape* to analyze the "multiple intersections of the times of culture and the socio-physical environment."[59] In this mode of analysis, she focuses on different kinds of rhythms and how they interact with each other; she describes the complexity and "interpenetration" of rhythms that may typically be seen as at odds with one another. By focusing on different scales and rhythms of modern timescapes, Adam aims to make visible some modes of time and place that have been rendered invisible by more dominant ones. In this book I work toward the same kind of analysis using the case of asthma care. As an environmental health disease, asthma is produced, triggered, and cared for through emplaced practices—embodied responses anchored in specific contexts—that lean into different kinds of rhythms, such as the rhythms of breathing, seasonal rhythms, the timing of paychecks, and exercise regimens.

In many of these instances, asthma sufferers not only use temporal rhythms and place-based knowledge to care for disordered breathing, but they also make *time* through care practices. Scholars have long argued that time is always made in one way or another, often through labor practices. María Puig de la Bellacasa has recently advanced the idea of making time for care time to describe specific soil care practices.[60] In the example of soil care, she shows that there are "a diversity of interdependent temporalities of beings and things at the heart of the predominant futuristic timescales of technoscientific expectations."[61] Care time brings in rhythms, temporalities, and patterns that may be devalued or even overridden in biomedicalized care practices. Ecological timescapes are one such example, and one particularly important for asthma care. The examples of asthma care described in this book show how a variety of temporalities converge, overlap, work together, and conflict in different contexts of breathing and disordered breathing.

Another mode of care necessary to situate the work of caring for asthma involves designing, building, and maintaining infrastructures.[62] Chronic care infrastructures, in particular, help to enable some kinds of care practices. Medical sociologist Henriette Langstrup uses the term *chronic care infrastructures* to describe the sociotechnical systems that enable treatment beyond the clinic.[63] These infrastructures, which include medications, biomedical standards, management guidelines, data, and assessment tools, enable care practices wherever patients travel, throughout everyday life. Chronic care infrastructures highlight the labor of care; the phrase emphasizes how the sociotechnical arrangements between the clinic and the world beyond support specific kinds of biomedical practices in relation to certain kinds of expertise, standards, and technologies. Chronic care infrastructures also demand participation from patients, who must utilize and maintain their relationships with the clinic through appointments, prescription refills, and illness tracking. Asthma care today depends more and more on the spatiotemporal arrangements of the home and the clinic, and all the places in between where breathers may need to care for their disease. Of course, access to chronic care infrastructures depends on health care access and medical insurance that can pay for such arrangements and their biomedical interventions.

Knowledge production and governance can be (should be) acts of care, too.[64] Care for asthma becomes a public matter, for example, because of the way respiratory health is connected to environmental conditions that must be governed. Asthma provides a very strong example of how care for environmental health must exceed the clinic, global markets, and private life.[65] Similar to the way in which chronic care infrastructures create and support particular modes of care, the concept of *carescapes* describes a web of care knit together with policy and organizational practices.[66] This approach to understanding asthma care looks at government policies and programs that are designed to address the asthma epidemic, including federally administered disease management guidelines, air pollution research and regulation, and health care for those otherwise unable to afford it.

There are many examples of public health carescapes that help people achieve asthma control.[67] Much of this work, however, has largely been geared toward cultivating and reinforcing individual care practices, such as pharmaceutical adherence, domestic cleaning regimens, and the tracking of pulmonary performance. As medical anthropologist Annemarie Mol has argued, "Citizenship requires us to control our bodies, to silence, or to discard them."[68] Public health carescapes become an important way to keep populations breathing so as to not overburden the national economy.[69] Increasingly these carescapes are directed toward supporting individual biomedical care practices.

The care enacted through infrastructures, policies, and government programs does not always address the specific, embodied, situated conditions of the problems identified, at least not directly. The way care is enacted always reflects ethical commitments. This is especially apparent in the work done by government, organizations, and research. My focus on care in this book should be read as a political orientation.[70] Scholarship on care points to power. Specifically, it asks, who cares, and how do we care? But it also asks, how does power afford different modes of care, where, and for whom?[71] In the case of disordered breathing, different modes of care emerge, for example, in relation to social determinants of health. The conditions of home and neighborhood environments, modes of transportation, types of work and where work is performed, access to health care, and social stigma—these are just a few of the dynamics that come into play as people care for asthma. People's ability to breathe freely also depends on privilege—for instance, whether they have time to relax, whether they are in the company of people they trust, and whether, in the long term, they have the resources to modify their lives to reduce exposures that trigger symptoms, now and in the future.[72] The ways that people enact care for asthma not only depend on power but can also augment or limit power. Tracing care across the sites described below helps to expose the unevenness of care tactics and also shows how breathing and its disorders track onto configurations of power and inequality.

The care work of the scholar who reflects on how a problem like the contemporary asthma epidemic is cared for must necessarily circulate through the spaces that constitute our cultural response.[73] My intention here is to contribute to the rich and always growing literature that documents "context-specific" and "perspective-dependent" forms of care.[74] By focusing on these different modes of care I hope to highlight what Michelle Murphy describes as "the layered and overlapping configurations that have materialized life in multiple and inconsistent ways over time and across space."[75]

A Multisited Ethnography

The research presented in this book was designed as a multisited ethnography tracing asthma care across sites of disease experience, environmental degradation, knowledge production, and public health work. The contrasting vignettes that opened this introduction provide a sense of how asthma traverses different scales, from the home as a site where individuals enact care to the public atmospheres that we collectively breathe. This book features other scales as well, from the global scale of climate change, with its impact on ecosystems, cities, and even interdisciplinary research, to the bedroom, the workplace, and the daily routines of asthmatics and caregivers. In the following chapters, I trace the relationships among discourse, practice, space, time, culture, economy, subjectivity, and various modes of knowing. Thinking of asthma care as an open system that, as Kim Fortun describes it, is "continually being reconstituted through the interaction of many scales, variables and forces" has allowed me to make sense of what asthma means in different contexts.[76]

I conducted the research for this book from March 2009 through August 2017, collecting data on the ground in seven U.S. cities. The sites

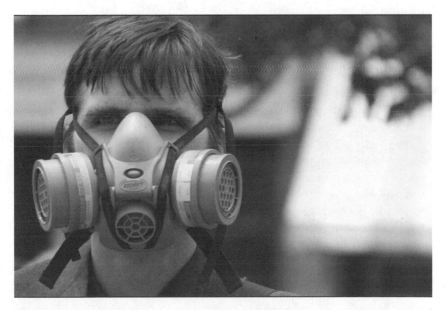

My earliest fieldwork was conducted with United Mountain Defense, a grassroots environmental justice organization based in Knoxville, Tennessee. I took this photograph of community organizer Matt Landon at a rally for clean air in August 2009.

of my participant observation included environmental justice rallies and public meetings hosted by nongovernmental organizations, science conferences and asthma care fund-raisers, and free asthma clinics in neighborhoods with asthma prevalence rates that far exceed the national average. I also worked closely with three organizations (one in Knoxville, Tennessee, for nine months, and two in Philadelphia for the last few years) that address local asthma epidemics through environmental justice work. I conducted two dozen interviews with staff members at eighteen organizations. Some of these were local, community-level organizations, others were state-level advocacy groups, and a handful were national or international in scope. The staff members interviewed were medical providers, community health workers, grassroots organizers, public health educators, and policy experts. I also conducted fifteen interviews with university-based scientists who received federal grants to investigate asthma and comorbid conditions; these interviews were conducted in summer 2015.

Most of the material described thus far provided background data that helped me to understand the context of asthma care today. The text is anchored by eighty-one interviews with people who have lived with asthma: twenty-two college students (ages eighteen to twenty-four, of whom three-quarters were women and two-thirds were white), twenty-one asthma sufferers who use the Buteyko breathing technique as a mode of care (ranging in age from late thirties to late sixties, of whom three-quarters were women and all were white), and thirty-eight other asthmatics whom I met through personal contacts over the course of conducting the research (ranging in age from twenty to sixty-seven, of whom all were middle- or working-class, about two-thirds were white, and just over half were men). The set of interviews is not representative of the U.S. asthma population, certainly not in terms of race and ethnicity.

My focus on asthma care practices and the interviews that followed began with a semester-long study of college students' perceptions of environment and health at Rensselaer Polytechnic Institute (RPI). Undertaken as part of a group project spearheaded by anthropologist Kim Fortun, who was teaching a class called Asthmatic Spaces, the study was organized around an online survey that was administered in April 2010. Our team collected more than a thousand responses, which led to twenty-two in-depth interviews with students with asthma. This set of interviews lent insight into how people with disordered breathing experience different climates, buildings, and seasons. Students who had lived their entire lives in the same residences or towns, for example, experienced changes when they moved to Upstate New York, where RPI is located. Some found that their symptoms increased, whereas for others the disease practically disappeared.

Many needed to adjust their asthma medications within their first year of attending RPI. Students who saw changes in their illness attributed them to housing conditions and to exposure to pollen and other seasonal variations that were unfamiliar to their bodies, as well as to lifestyle changes, which are a central feature of the transition to college.

Students spoke of nonadherence to medication regimens and even expressed outright hostility toward pharmaceuticals in these interviews. Having transitioned out of domains where parents or guardians may have helped them take daily controller medications or insisted that they do so, some students felt free to abandon these regimens; they judged that they could manage symptoms on the fly, so to speak. For some, changes in their daily routines, or lack of routines, made it difficult for them to remember to take medications. Others no longer experienced asthma symptoms at all and stopped taking medications completely, transitions that may or may not have taken place under the guidance of doctors. Several, however, maintained the exact same regimens that they had been adhering to for years.

Changes in chronic care infrastructures constituted yet another theme within this set of interviews. As newly minted adults, these college students had begun to navigate the health care system on their own, which often meant that they had visited the college's student health clinic. Of the many insights gained from this set of interviews, place emerged as a central component, if not a determinant, of disease experience and care, not only on a daily basis but also in terms of such major life decisions as those concerning human relationships and housing. The dynamics of place were enmeshed in the creative, resistant, compliant, and at times difficult decisions that the students with asthma made.

The RPI study was followed by more than thirty-eight in-depth interviews with asthmatics whom I met at field sites over the next eight years: neighbors, students, shop owners, community organizers, engineers, professional staff members at the nonprofits where I conducted fieldwork, scientists, parents of asthmatics, and friends of friends. Whenever I met someone with asthma, if it was appropriate to the conversation, I tried to ask for an interview. (If I have learned anything over the course of this project, it is that many, many people have direct experience with asthma; at times I have suspected that national prevalence rates of the disease may be very conservative.) Some of those I interviewed lived with mild asthma, others with moderate and well-controlled asthma, and still others with severe asthma; a few suffered from asthma in its uncontrolled form. Almost all of those interviewed were diagnosed after 1985, when national attention turned toward the asthma epidemic, particularly in children.[77]

More than half of the interviewees had been diagnosed nearly a decade ago, often while under the care of parents or guardians. Several who were over the age of fifty had been diagnosed in the past twenty years but believed they had suffered from undiagnosed asthma since childhood. For those who did remember diagnosis and early patient–health care provider interaction, there were clear differences between their experiences and the treatments that are professionally espoused and recommended today. Trends in asthma treatment and diagnosis, of course, have changed significantly in the past twenty-five years. Patient education is undoubtedly better, for example, although there are still wide variations in how general practitioners handle asthma management.

The people I interviewed described their asthma attacks in visceral detail. They told me about midnight nebulizer treatments and trips to the emergency room; halted sports games and inhalers on loan; the smells of chemicals, smoke, and perfume; itchy throats and premonitions before wheezing begins. My interviews with asthma sufferers covered their medication use, environmental control practices, quality of life, interactions with the medical establishment, everyday perceptions, and theories of disease. The stories that emerged from these interviews provided me with a rich sense of how asthma structures both daily life and life trajectories through the experience of place and environment, in ways inflected by race, class, and gender.

For some of the asthmatics I spoke with, however, the disease did more than structure life: it completely hijacked it. While the majority of people diagnosed with asthma have either a mild version of the disease or a variant that responds to standard medications, a small percentage of people live with severe asthma. A person may be diagnosed with severe asthma if high doses of inhaled corticosteroids and other medications are needed to keep symptoms under control or if the person's symptoms cannot be controlled even with high doses of standard medications.[78] I began to learn more specifically about the experiences of severe asthmatics in 2010 when I read an article in the *New York Times* that described a "natural" therapy for asthma.[79]

Learning about the Buteyko breathing technique (BBT), and the international community of breathing educators who teach people how to use it, significantly deepened my perspective on asthma. My study of the breathing educators' community began with a two-month internship at a clinic in New York's Hudson Valley. This was followed by interviews with breathing educators, participant observation in one-on-one client sessions, and attendance at weekend workshops and the annual meetings of the Buteyko Breathing Educators Association. Because many breathing educators are themselves asthma sufferers, my research with this community of practice gave me further insight into the disease experience and the dynamics of care. Some of the Buteyko breathing educators I met had been severely asthmatic before learning BBT; their experience with pharmaceutical regimens had been unsuccessful, or the amount of medication they needed for daily disease management seemed excessive. Those I interviewed told me that their practice of BBT, and related lifestyle changes, had dramatically improved their quality of life. In many cases, they were now incorporating BBT into their existing professional lives or were teaching BBT classes as a second career. The group included respiratory therapists, bodyworkers, voice therapists, hygienists, and others working in health care professions where breathing exercises and knowledge of breathing techniques could easily be incorporated.

Despite their own experiences with BBT and the premises of the tradition, the members of the Buteyko breathing educator community with whom I spoke had little interest in challenging the medical establishment or the pharmaceutical industry. Rather, they focused their efforts on making a complementary method of disease management visible by recentering attention on breathing patterns and techniques. They hoped to connect with struggling asthmatics and other patient populations who suffered from disordered breathing. For this reason, some Buteyko educators reached out to local medical professionals and clinics, with varying degrees of success. Many physicians have never heard of BBT; outside Russia, where the technique was first developed in the 1950s, merely a dozen clinical studies have been conducted on the method. A few of the senior Buteyko breathing educators I interviewed had attempted to secure legitimacy for the tradition in the medical sciences by establishing collaborations with university scientists to conduct clinical studies. In a context where most research dollars flow to treatments that advance biomedical technologies, however, these activities found little traction. Nor is BBT easy to implement—the practice is challenging and time-consuming, a poor fit in a culture that values quick remedies involving little effort. My ongoing research with the Buteyko breathing educator community added complexity to my understanding of asthma, revealing the hegemony of biomedical perspectives at multiple levels and from new angles.

Around the time I learned of the community of Buteyko breathing educators, I also began hearing about Asthmapolis, a mobile phone application that garnered headlines in 2010 when it promised to geocode asthma attacks. Health apps for smartphones exemplify the kind of transformation seen in the age of biomedicalization; they are firmly entrenched in dominant modes of pharmaceutical-based care but are a form of personal technology that shifts ways of thinking about and enacting care using data infrastructures. As the smartphone market has grown, so too has the market for health-focused apps, including apps for disease management. The development of Asthmapolis emerged from a collaboration between David Van Sickle, a public health professor at the University of Wisconsin, and a group of engineering students. Although not the first asthma-focused mobile app in the market, Asthmapolis was noteworthy because of its use of a GPS sensor that fit onto a rescue inhaler. Each time the inhaler was used, time and location information would be sent to the user's account. The aim was to help breathers track how often they experienced asthma symptoms, and where. Asthmapolis users could also opt to share their data with their health care providers to give them a fuller, more accurate picture of their illness. That, however, was something that any mobile asthma app in the emerging market was poised to do. What made Asthmapolis unique was its ability to crowdsource symptom event data. This function enabled researchers to analyze data on the locations and times of attacks against other data sets, such as air quality readings; researchers embraced the app's potential to contribute public health value through personal technologies.

In 2014, four years after Asthmapolis made headlines, the company changed its name to Propeller Health, signaling a move to expand its user base to include people with other chronic respiratory conditions as well as those with asthma. Van Sickle, now CEO of a company that had raised millions of dollars for research and product development, had succeeded in getting the project out of the university and into the field; studies were in process, and patients could sign up to participate as Propeller Health gathered patient data. But by now, the company's app, now called Propeller, had been joined by hundreds of other apps for asthma care. The field was brimming with sleek mobile platforms developed by all kinds of organizations—clinics and hospitals, governments, tech start-ups, and, of course, pharmaceutical companies. From December 2014 through August 2015, I analyzed more than three hundred mobile asthma apps, assessing how their designs and algorithms added value to existing care protocols.[80] Were these personal technologies shifting disease discourse and care practices? My interviews with representatives from organizations developing mobile asthma apps reflected the incredible complexity of the U.S. health care system and the characteristics of biomedicalization in process.[81]

The final layer of ethnographic fieldwork that shaped this book took place over four years, 2013–17, while I was working on environmental health projects in Philadelphia.[82] As mentioned previously, asthma is a problem in Philadelphia for a number of reasons, including poor air quality, an aging built environment, high poverty rates, and variable access to health care. If you work in health care, education, or the environmental sector in Philadelphia, you hear about asthma. By many accounts, Philadelphia is a space that is becoming increasingly unbreathable. One of the ways I have learned about Philadelphia's asthma epidemic, and the carescapes that help manage it, is through the Climate, Health, and Home project, which exemplifies emergent cross-sectoral collaborations among environmental nonprofits, health management organizations, science educators, and local government. In this leg of my fieldwork, I was a core collaborator as much as a participant observer, assisting not only with data collection and analysis but also with workshop design and facilitation. Over the four-year period, twelve collaborators from nine organizations ran a total of nine workshops attended by more than two hundred community members and twenty-four staff members working in Philadelphia's health care sector. As the name would suggest, the Climate, Health, and Home project is specifically designed to educate people about and develop strategies to address the effects of climate change on the home front. Data from this piece of fieldwork include information gathered through participant observation in project workshops as well as in meetings and events involving our project team and the many other stakeholder groups actively working at the intersection of health and climate in Philadelphia.

One of the limitations of this book is a lack of accounts from inside the clinic itself, between doctor and patient. While I include testimonials of people's experiences with doctors in medical settings, it is not my aim to examine the relationships or encounters between patients and health care providers. There is no doubt that patient–provider interactions are hugely important for illness experience and treatment practices; indeed, these relationships have figured prominently in medical sociology and anthropology. But while the absence of patient–provider accounts might be interpreted as a flaw in this study, I have come to embrace it as a strength. This volume documents disease experiences and care practices beyond health care sites, on the streets, in people's homes, as they travel and exercise, in their everyday lives. The lived experiences and perspectives conveyed through the interviews presented here have largely been rendered invisible and therefore unstudied in the social and medical sciences, which have focused on other scales of analysis.[83] There are a number of reasons for this invisibility: care happens outside the clinic because of a lack of health insurance or the desire to save money; illness becomes normalized over time, particularly after a person has lived with the disease for decades; asthma is stigmatized, owing to cultural legacies that extend back centuries; changes in life status alter access to health care and engagement with medical providers; changes in life status alter the disease experience itself;

cultural beliefs about health and medicine are not fully explored; and, finally, the very nature of asthma as an intermittent, variable disease condition shapes our social engagement with it. These and other dynamics that render asthma invisible are discussed in depth in the pages to come.

Snapshots of Asthma Care

The next five chapters depict scenes of life with asthma and perspectives on the disease through the interplay of different modes of care, shown through different practices and scales of health care. Chapters 1 through 3 are empirically anchored by asthmatics' experiences to show how the disease is understood biomedically and environmentally, as well as how disordered breathing is managed with and without medication. These chapters lean into asthmatic subjectivity and care practices, but they do so against the backdrop of human–nonhuman interaction, biomedicalization, and the discursive work performed by organizations that have a stake in asthma care. Chapters 1 and 2 draw primarily from the interviews I conducted with asthma sufferers, historical and literary texts, and peer-reviewed literature and public health documents. Chapter 3 is a case study focusing on the Buteyko breathing technique and its life in the international community of practice. The final two chapters present asthma in emerging care contexts — the mobile health marketplace and public health approaches to climate change in Philadelphia. These chapters highlight the political, economic, and technological dynamics of asthma care differently than earlier chapters, with more emphasis on the roles of markets, policy, and populations. Taken together, chapters 4 and 5 provide a sense of how asthma, as an object of care, matters on a broad scale: how a panoply of approaches, individually and collectively configured, respond to the slow and uneven violence that makes the world increasingly unbreathable.

CHAPTER ONE

Attuning to Asthma in Time and Place

I don't have full-blown asthma, I have never needed shots and I don't have a maintenance inhaler, but I have exercise-induced asthma and I have had asthma attacks at various points in my life. They generally only last for a month and I have only had three of those. The exercise-induced asthma I was diagnosed with in sixth grade, so I was around eleven, when I really started doing sports. My chest would sort of seize up and I wouldn't be able to breathe. So I went to the doctor. But I would never get to the point of passing out or going to the ER. But I would have to go to the sideline and sit down. Eventually I would be able to catch my breath. So I got albuterol and I would do that before exercise, but I have had to do that pretty much my whole life. I was told to use it like, twice before exercise. Just two puffs. Like fifteen minutes to a half hour before exercise. And then if during exercise I started having trouble breathing, I could do one more. It seems to work. It's not really an asthma attack because I have friends that have real asthma, so I don't want to compare it to that, but if I have to use my inhaler and I'm exercising too hard, I sort of get a shortness of breath and it feels like each breath isn't doing anything. Before I can get anything, it's gone. So it's like I'm breathing really hard, but it's very shallow. It feels like it can't catch.

An asthmatic in his mid-twenties, Shaun told a story that was both similar to and different from those I heard in my interviews with other asthmatics. It was different in the details of Shaun's experiences and his description of breathlessness, but similar in his age of disease onset, his use of medication, and his somatic awareness. His distancing of the disease he experiences from "real asthma" is a common theme in conversations I have had with breathers who have been diagnosed with the disease. Over the course of our interview, Shaun detailed three forms of asthma, only two of which he named as such, asthma. This is not surprising, since Shaun has received only one diagnosis for his condition: exercise-induced asthma (EIA). In Shaun's mind, he is not a real asthmatic with "full-blown asthma" because his experience of disordered breathing is limited to specific situations— when he is exercising and on two occasions while he was at work, which he considered isolated events. Real asthma, in his account, involves emergency room visits, passing out, a daily medication regimen, and allergy shots; these are all signals of chronicity, severity, and sensitivity that Shaun does not personally associate with his condition.

At the time he was diagnosed with EIA, nearly fifteen years ago, Shaun experienced breathing difficulty only when he was playing sports, a very delimited context. His doctor prescribed albuterol as a preventive measure and instructed him to use it before physical activity. Albuterol is a short-acting beta-2 adrenergic agonist (SABA) drug, a bronchodilator that relaxes and opens airways that have narrowed. People with asthma use albuterol inhalers, known as rescue inhalers, when respiratory symptoms emerge—when they experience shortness of breath, wheezing, chest constriction, or coughing, for example. Bronchodilators have been prescribed universally for asthma attacks since the 1970s.[1] People diagnosed with EIA, however, often use albuterol prior to engaging in physical activity, as a preventive medication rather than in response to respiratory symptoms.

Shaun's preventive use of a rescue inhaler had been the extent of his treatment regimen until, years later, shortly after high school, he had an attack that was not related to physical activity:

> I had to go to a doctor once, but this was a different type of asthma attack. But it might have been something different. I was working in a theater and I got exposed to some dust and I have no idea what the dust was, but I instantly couldn't breathe and it felt like one of my other—the same thing—so I sat down and just couldn't breathe. And it wasn't to the point of passing out, but I immediately went to go see a doctor. Someone actually drove me there. They gave me an inhaler on the spot. So I took that and had to take that for like a month. That happened like twice when I was working there. Not sure what it was.

Shaun experienced this second form of asthma as isolated attacks limited to whatever was in the dust at the theater where he worked. The attacks at the theater were more severe and instantaneous than the breathlessness Shaun experienced during physical activity. The symptom was familiar, if more immediate and forceful, but it seemed out of place with his diagnosed disease context, EIA. Following the first asthma attack at the theater, an urgent care doctor prescribed Shaun an inhaled controller medication that he used twice a day for a month. Controller inhalers, also known as maintenance inhalers, are prescribed when a patient has uncontrolled, severe, or allergic asthma—that is, when symptoms emerge in a range of contexts several times a week or with a spontaneous severity that could be life threatening. Controller inhalers deliver anti-inflammatory medications to control airway sensitivity and inflammation. These kinds of medications are intended to make patients less reactive to environmental triggers.

Later in his interview, Shaun described a possible third form of asthma, although he did not name it as such:

> It's so weird. I got really bad allergies in the spring every year that I
> lived in Maine. Moved to Boston—fine. Moved back to Maine—
> horrible. Then here I haven't had allergies this season at all. I get it
> really bad in the spring and the fall too. Probably right around now.
> I would be sick for like a month. I would usually get put on medication
> for whatever it caused. Like, I have had bronchial infections with a lot
> of coughing and I have had sinus infections. The bronchial infections,
> I actually got those for three out of the four years that I was in Maine
> and I would always get it at the same time. But it was always like, I
> would have a sore throat for a week and have a cough, but the cough
> was really persistent and then after three weeks—I don't know why
> I wouldn't go right in. This was usually like right around now. I would
> go in and they would be like, oh, you have bronchitis. Then I would get
> an antibiotic or something, I'm not sure what it was. And cough
> medicine, like the codeine stuff. That was usually why I would go in,
> because I couldn't sleep because I would be coughing all night.

Although Shaun connected both EIA and the attacks at the theater (even if hesitantly) to asthma, it was only when I asked if he had allergies that he brought up this third case of disordered breathing. I was surprised that Shaun's doctor had not connected his seasonal allergies, which also required medication (antibiotics and prescription cough medicine), to his asthma diagnosis. Shaun's narrative mirrors clinical and anecdotal definitions of allergic asthma in its seasonal manifestation. In my reading of Shaun's case, the tell is his persistent cough, which he often experienced at night.

Until relatively recently, doctors and scientists believed asthma was primarily an allergic disease, in the same category as hay fever and eczema. But asthma is different from allergies, if not always separate from them. The term *asthma* applies specifically to difficulties with breathing, and in ways that are not always connected to allergies. Allergies and asthma have a complex, entangled relationship, as evidenced by the use of such terms as *allergic asthma* and *atopic asthma*. *Atopy* refers to immunoglobulin E–mediated reactions to environmental matter, from dust, dander, and pollen to peanuts. Today, the scientific literature recognizes at least half a dozen asthma phenotypes, several of which—including exercise-induced asthma—have nothing to do with allergies.[2] Allergy narratives nevertheless dominate most histories of asthma, and biographies of famous asthmatics are punctuated by the cyclical nature of seasonal allergies such as hay fever.[3] The relationship between allergies and asthma, however, is far from fully parsed out by scientists.

Reading Shaun's narrative against the scientific and historical literature, his case strikes me as a classic one of allergy-related asthma, albeit possibly undiagnosed and undertreated. This is a strange suggestion to make in a time when many believe that illnesses in general are overdiagnosed and overtreated.[4] Then again, as I will show, asthma can go undetected—that is one of its trademarks. When I asked Shaun if he had ever been tested for allergies, he told me he had not; seasonal allergies ran in his family, so he felt he knew what they were and how to deal with them. Plus, he only ever had problems while living in Maine, and then only for two or three months out of the year. He never experienced seasonal allergy symptoms when living in Massachusetts, New York, or New Jersey. His need for medical care was isolated to particular places and times, for the most part. In his mind, this was not a chronic condition. Daily medication seemed unnecessary given the cyclical and emplaced nature of his breathing disorder. In Shaun's view, all he really needed was an albuterol inhaler to use preventively before physical activity. His other experiences were isolated events rather than signals of a persistent underlying condition.

How asthma sufferers develop their own classification systems for asthma is one of the focal points of this chapter.[5] The classifications that people use may build on medical diagnoses and treatment protocols, but they may also include other factors, such as sensations, breathing rhythms, and emplaced knowledge. One reason for this is that asthma is an environmental health condition; symptoms emerge in particular places and at particular times. Paying attention to timescapes and environmental qualities in relation to breathing helps people with asthma manage their disease.

Asthma is a heterogeneous and variable disease, too. It looks different from one person to the next, as well as in the same person over time and place. Shaun, for example, had seasonal allergies, but only in Maine. Yet his allergies produced breathing problems too (a nighttime cough) that would not go away on their own. For Shaun, the differences in his experiences of disordered breathing—the feelings and contexts—were meaningful. Breathlessness in exercise and a swift inability to breathe in the theater were asthma; coughing during allergy season was not. Both are examples of disordered breathing and illness, but in very different contexts with differences in symptoms. And Shaun relied heavily on his doctor's diagnosis of EIA for his own meaning-making and care practices. Without the name "asthma" attached to the two other cases of disordered breathing, he was not sure how his symptoms all fit together.

The people I interviewed for this project usually had two reasons they agreed to talk with me: they wanted to share their disease experience, and they wanted answers. Representations of asthma in media accounts, cultural imaginaries, and management protocols suggest that asthma is a singular, simple disease in which breathers experience attacks of breathlessness. Given these representations, it is easy to view asthma as a closed case, easily treatable. In daily life, the clinic, and the lab, however, asthma is much more heterogeneous and open. In this chapter I show how the heterogeneity of asthma plays out in two contexts: in the experiences and knowledge of those who live with disordered breathing, and in medical documents, including diagnostic guidelines and peer-reviewed publications. Placing these different ways of conceptualizing asthma side by side reveals how different epistemic standpoints lead to similar conclusions within very different modes of knowing. Both standpoints reflect a language for asthma characterized by manifold heterogeneity, a proliferation of disease dimensions anchored by affect, time, and place.

What's in a Name?

More than twenty years ago, journalist Tim Brookes went looking for answers to the same questions that troubled the breathers I interviewed. In his early thirties at the time, Brookes had an asthma attack that caught him off guard and nearly killed him. Like Shaun in the theater, Brookes was not exactly sure what triggered the attack, despite the fact that he had lived with asthma for decades. "The first line of treatment is avoidance. But avoidance of what? The asthmatic is doomed to gnaw on the event until he finds a clue, a cause. What did he do? What did he eat? What did he breathe?"[6] The life-threatening attack made him realize just how little he knew about the disease. How could he care for his asthma without a better understanding of how it works?

Brookes wrote a memoir, *Catching My Breath: An Asthmatic Explores His Illness*, investigating his long struggle with atopic asthma. One of the many crucial things he learned during his investigation is that asthma is episodic, and also much more than the symptom event. It does not consist only of the attack; the attack is just the tipping point of the disease. Asthma is always there, whether the asthmatic has symptoms or not. "Once you understand this," he writes, "you recognize the dormant phase, the buildup with its drop in pulmonary function, and see the acute phase as merely the culmination, the manifestation, the word made flesh."[7]

The idea of a one-to-one relationship between stimulus and reaction, trigger and attack, is common in representations of asthma, but it is also misleading. It leaves out the layers and the relationships that make asthma so difficult to know. The linearity that Brookes relays—dormancy, buildup, and drop in functioning—may not actually characterize underlying disease mechanisms. And the breather may certainly not feel these steps. Both Shaun and Brookes experienced severe, instantaneous attacks that seemingly came out of nowhere, catching them off guard. These attacks were different from the subtler symptoms they were familiar with, the smaller experiences of asthma that emerge in everyday or cyclical contexts. This is the crux of what both of them wanted to know: Where did *that* (attack) come from? What caused it? Was it as simple as the triggering object, the one Brookes searched for following his near-death experience? Was there something in the environment that made the attack different from other, more common, low-grade asthmatic events? Or was there something going on inside the body, something happening in the immune system that made the body more reactive to the surrounding environment? How exactly did the entanglement of body and environment produce this attack? And what did time have to do with it?[8]

For both Shaun and Brookes, these asthma attacks were different kinds of events from what they typically experienced as asthma. Yet, when asked, many asthmatics will describe different kinds of asthma that inhabit their bodies. Brookes himself had a classification system built on his experiences in different contexts. This involved sensing where symptoms emerged in the body, how they felt, their force and speed. Cultural anthropologist Kathleen Stewart has termed such awareness *atmospheric attunement,* our sentient attention to the matter of everyday life as it emerges. The crux of atmospheric attunement is that our attention is focused on the "qualities, rhythms, forces, relations, and movements" of our situation in the world, in a place and with time.[9]

Brookes's memoir includes a list of different forms of asthma, reflecting his attunement to shifting patterns and feelings in his body—when and where disordered breathing emerged:

- a sudden overwhelming, massive attack like last November's, with enormous secretions of watery mucus;
- a gentle evening creep, with no apparent tightness or tension in the chest at all;
- moist seasonal wheezing accompanied by symptoms of hay fever;
- tension localized in the chest, with virtually no wheeze at all and no apparent grounding in anxiety (sometimes asthma disguises itself so well that I don't even realize it's there; it feels as if I'm slightly on edge, and I surprise myself by catching the echo of a faint wheeze);
- tension in the throat and neck, especially at times of anxiety;
- exercise-induced asthma, a gasping, laboring breathing (which I don't seem to have suffered from for at least fifteen years);
- cold-air asthma, with an attendant heaviness in the shoulders.[10]

The items in this laundry list of types of asthma are distinguished by time, space, feeling, force, and affect. Brookes notes how he senses changes in breathing rhythms or feelings in his lungs, shifts in his body—but always in relation to places or times. For Brookes, and others like him, asthma is much more than an attack of breathlessness. It means different modes of disorder, connected to particular sensations and emotions, sounds, times of day and year, activities, and environmental conditions—an entanglement of multiple kinds of things known through attunement. The ability to differentiate matter and force in breathing in space is precisely the kind of emplaced knowing that anchors asthma care practices for many breathers. Asthmatic attunement involves attention to material differences and their affects, which inform caring responses.

Not all asthma attacks are created equal. Some are indeed events of attack, but others seem not to be events at all, but rather states that one can subtly slip into. Kevin, a forty-year-old white man from a working-class family living outside Boston, described three types of asthma that he experiences. In doing so, he referred to both how his breath feels and the conditions under which his disordered breathing emerges:

> I know I have sort of typical allergy seasons in spring for example, right now, and I find that my asthma will be more of a nuisance asthma. I very rarely have heavy, really crazy, asthma attacks anymore. It's mostly a nuisance asthma. Meaning that you will have low-level breathing difficulties. Like, you can feel yourself wheezing. It comes in two ways—one would be lack of breath and I will be like, oh, I'm having a hard time breathing. Or I kind of feel myself wheezing and that's a sign. Or if I'm feeling sick and I start feeling crackling in my lungs. That's another sign. Each of those are signs of three different things. Feeling

difficulty breathing is something that feels as though it's an immediate problem. The wheezing kind of thing is more like a nuisance asthma and the crackling is like, oh crap, I'm getting a lung infection. For the most part, I have noticed that it's less intense than what it was when I was younger.

Kevin was diagnosed at age eleven after an exercise-induced asthma attack, at which point his doctor identified him as an allergic asthmatic. It was a clear case, Kevin told me, since he had eczema, seasonal allergies, and sensitivity to animal dander. Disordered breathing was an intensified version of his embodied reaction to environmental matter; Kevin, his parents, and his doctor became aware of the severity of Kevin's asthma when he had an attack while running around at a birthday party. That was more than twenty-five years ago, however, and over time, Kevin's asthma had become less intense. He attributed this to his ability to be "more aware of what environmental hazards there are" around him.

By staying attuned to the changes in his breath and a feeling in his lungs, Kevin had developed an emplaced knowledge of the contexts and conditions that trigger his asthma. He had translated his asthmatic attunement into a classification system in which he associated particular kinds of environmental matter, times of year, and relationships with different symptoms, with different kinds of asthma. While this kind of system may work well for individuals like Kevin and Brookes—indeed, Kevin later told me that his classification system allowed him to manage his asthma so that it had become less intense than it was when he was growing up, a subject I will return to later—such attuned knowledge systems, or "worldings," in Stewart's language, have been difficult to translate to medical arenas.[11] This is not for a lack of effort on the part of biomedical researchers, however.[12]

A review of publications on asthma produced by public health organizations and medical associations reveals definitions of asthma that are not only broad but also inconclusive and open-ended. The most current definition at the time of this writing, and the one that likely carries the most weight internationally, comes from the Global Initiative for Asthma (GINA), a public health collaboration anchored by the National Heart, Lung, and Blood Institute (NHLBI, part of the U.S. National Institutes of Health) and the World Health Organization. Established in 1993 in response to growing awareness of the global asthma epidemic, GINA reviews asthma research and publishes international guidelines for diagnosis and management. Its 2018 updated report on asthma management and prevention provides the following description:

Asthma is characterized by variable symptoms of wheeze, shortness of breath, chest tightness and/or cough, and by variable expiratory airflow limitation. Both symptoms and airflow limitation characteristically vary over time and in intensity. These variations are often triggered by factors such as exercise, allergen or irritant exposure, change in weather, or viral respiratory infections.

Symptoms and airflow limitation may resolve spontaneously or in response to medication, and may sometimes be absent for weeks or months at a time. On the other hand, patients can experience episodic flare-ups (exacerbations) of asthma that may be life-threatening and carry a significant burden to patients and the community. Asthma is usually associated with airway hyperresponsiveness to direct or indirect stimuli, and with chronic airway inflammation. These features usually persist, even when symptoms are absent or lung function is normal, but may normalize with treatment.[13]

In the first paragraph, describing components of the disease, the word "variable" appears twice, along with "vary" and "variation." Symptoms are variable. Airflow limitation is variable. Intensity and duration are variable. Triggers are variable. This wording suggests that the name *asthma* is doing a lot of work, as it is broadly applied to many symptoms and situations.

The second paragraph quoted above, states that symptoms may clear up on their own, but they may also return spontaneously, and with life-threatening intensity. The disease is visible *and* invisible; a person may or may not have symptoms, but key features of asthma "usually persist, even when symptoms are absent or lung function is normal." Asthma is not only variable but also undetectable; GINA's description states clearly that the disease is present even without the kinds of embodied signs that allow people like Brookes and Kevin to know their disease and care for it. Pulmonary performance tests that measure lung function cannot guarantee detection either.

This description additionally suggests that symptoms may be associated with direct stimuli or indirect stimuli, like exercise or stress. In other words, sometimes there is a clear relationship—the presence of a cat and the onset of wheezing, or damp moldy air and chest tightness—but in many cases, asthma attacks appear out of thin air. Both GINA's description of asthma and the reflections of asthma sufferers suggest a condition that is unpredictable. In light of this kind of manifold heterogeneity, where a proliferation of unpredictable dynamics conspires to produce disordered breathing, asthmatic attunement—a mode of being present that contextualizes sensation based on past experience and current situation—makes sense as a foundation for care for a disease that has many material variations and temporal layers.

Of course, there has also been a movement among researchers to develop a more nuanced, evidenced-based classification system to reflect asthma's heterogeneity. The GINA report continues its description of asthma with an emerging list of phenotypes:

> Asthma is a heterogeneous disease, with different underlying disease processes. Recognizable clusters of demographic, clinical and/or pathophysiological characteristics are often called "asthma phenotypes." In patients with more severe asthma, some phenotype-guided treatments are available. However, to date, no strong relationship has been found between specific pathological features and particular clinical patterns or treatment responses. More research is needed to understand the clinical utility of phenotypic classification in asthma.[14]

The report then lists "some of the most common" phenotypes: allergic asthma, non-allergic asthma, late-onset asthma, asthma with fixed airflow limitation, and asthma with obesity.[15] Other asthma phenotype models are more extensive. Phenotypes are defined as collections of characteristics that are clinically observable and can include, as is the case with asthma, collections of self-reported symptoms and illness narratives. An NHLBI document lists nine asthma phenotypes in three categories: phenotypes based on triggers, phenotypes based on clinical presentation, and phenotypes based on inflammatory markers.[16] Some phenotypes appear in multiple categories. In this model, exercise-induced asthma is a trigger-based phenotype as well as a phenotype in clinical presentation. Of the phenotype classification systems I have reviewed, all place allergic asthma at the top of the phenotype list, and all note that allergic asthma is the most common among the variants of asthma.

None of the phenotype models proposed—indeed, none of the phenotypes themselves—have been formally accepted by leading public health organizations such as GINA or by international research communities. An effort to change that is currently in the works, however. Sally Wenzel, a leading expert on asthma phenotypes and director of the University of Pittsburgh Asthma Institute, has explained that the reason no phenotype has been wholeheartedly accepted by the scientific community is that none of the proposed phenotypes have met all the definitional requirements of phenotype naming:

> The definition of a true phenotype (or endotype) requires a unifying and consistent natural history, consistent clinical and physiological characteristics, an underlying pathobiology with identifiable biomarkers

and genetics and a predictable response to general and specific therapies. . . . No present system of subgrouping achieves all the requirements for a true phenotype or endotype. In addition, there are a number of co-morbidities and confounders that have been identified that can alter asthma phenotypes.[17]

Asthma's complexity has overwhelmed medical efforts to create a standard definition and coherent classification system based on genetic understandings of disease. The literature on phenotypes does include some of the same elements that breathers use to identify and name their variants of asthma, specifically natural history and physiological characteristics, but current research on phenotypes also works to layer in molecular elements that are inaccessible to the average breather. Thus, phenotype definitions cast asthma in a language that is very different from the language Brookes

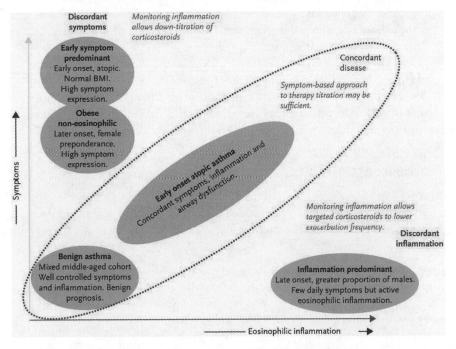

This illustration of different asthma phenotypes and the relationships among them indicates how the disease is characterized temporally and by specific kinds of symptoms, severity, and inflammation. Originally published in Clementine Bostantzoglou, Vicky Delimpoura, Konstantinos Samitas, Eleftherios Zervas, Frank Kanniess, and Mina Gaga, "Clinical Asthma Phenotypes in the Real World: Opportunities and Challenges," *Breathe* 11 (2015): 186–93. http://breathe .ersjournals.com/content/11/3/186.

uses in his list of asthma types. Somewhere along the path to classifying asthma's different forms, the emphasis on biomarkers and genetic dynamics renders invisible the importance and usefulness of attunement in everyday asthma care. Faith and investment in pharmaceutical treatments for asthma are backed, of course, by the success of controller medications, which have helped many people manage their disease.

In 1994, when *Catching My Breath* came out, only five years had passed since the asthma epidemic captured national headlines, garnering political and scientific attention. Brookes at the time surely assumed that answers to his biggest question—What exactly is asthma?—would be forthcoming, given the numbers of newly funded research programs aiming to address the epidemic. Yet in more than two decades of research—in the clinic, in animal models, in homes and neighborhoods, cross-referencing public health and environmental data as well as data from pharmaceutical trials on biologic applications—and with billions spent globally, the definition of asthma has only widened further. Inroads have been made, of course, but rather than reducing the number of theories of pathology, research programs have multiplied asthma further. Despite the challenges that Wenzel identifies, research on potential phenotype classification continues (indeed, Wenzel is pioneering this growing movement), particularly given the hope that through identification of biomarkers and genetic elements associated with asthma, more specific, personalized treatments can be developed.[18]

Diagnosing Disease

A registered nurse for more than thirty years, Brenda, age fifty-five, had witnessed the evolving ways in which asthma is classified and the impacts of those changes on clinical practice and education. She had also experienced the changes firsthand:

> I have asthma that is a little bit exertional and a lot if I get an upper respiratory infection. I don't consider myself a chronic asthmatic, but I do realize that I have to be very conscious if I get a cold, to be aware of where that is going. It's interesting, I always had problems as a kid but I wasn't diagnosed until my late forties, mid-forties. And I went through that my whole life until my mid-forties, and the thing that sort of turned the corner—it kept getting worse every time I would get a cold, it would be harder and harder for me to get over the cough. And then one evening I started laughing and I couldn't stop the coughing and I couldn't get my breath. I went to my doctor and she said to me, you have asthma. I was like, oh no, I don't. You don't get asthma at forty-seven, or whatever I was. She said, that's what you have. At that

point I was wheezing a little and now I know that when that tightness
happens, that that is what it is. Okay, no big deal, millions of people
get on with their life. But not exertional. No, I could walk but I often
get out of breath walking and maybe four years ago I had a cardiac
stress test, just because when you are fifty, you are supposed to have
that, the whole bit. I go in, the technician says, do you have asthma?
I said, only when I have a cold. They had to stop the test because I
couldn't breathe. And the woman goes, you have exertional asthma
also. So I think part of it is that as I get older, I do recognize that it
comes into my life in different ways, but it is certainly—I wouldn't say
that it impinges on anything. . . . I was sort of appalled at being told
that I had asthma and partly because my experience or my image of it
was much more debilitating than my personal experience was.

Time came up in the way Brenda framed her disease, and also in the manner her disordered breathing came to be diagnosed the second time
around. Time is a key element not only in asthmatic attunement, and by
extension care, but in clinical diagnosis as well. Brenda's response to being
told that she had asthma, "Oh no, I don't. You don't get asthma at forty-
seven," derived in part from entrenched cultural representations of what
a person with asthma looks like. Historically, representations of asthma
have featured feeble, sickly children who need their inhalers to do anything.[19] Today's media representations extend this imagery to adults as
well, sending messages that clash with the self-perceptions of those who
see themselves as healthy.[20] Brenda and Shaun both assumed asthma to be
a much more debilitating and severe disease than what they personally
experienced. And like many others I interviewed, Brenda believed asthma
to be a disease that starts in childhood; it is not something adults develop.
These views reflect the fact that for most of the twentieth century, the
clinical and scientific focus of asthma research in the United States was on
children with allergic asthma.

For decades, allergic asthma dominated not only pathophysiological
definitions, research trajectories, and pharmaceutical development but also
clinical conduct.[21] And one of the defining features of the allergic asthma
phenotype is that it begins during childhood.[22] The scientific and clinical
models that linked asthma and allergies were so strong that it seemed im-
plausible for adults without allergies to have asthma, as in Brenda's case.
Nevertheless, Brenda is part of a growing population: individuals—most
of whom are women—who experience disordered breathing in the absence
of allergies.[23]

As Brenda's story conveys, she likely developed asthma as a teenager,
but doctors at that time were not diagnosing asthma in cases that presented

as hers did. Growing up in rural New York in the 1960s and 1970s, Brenda received an annual diagnosis of bronchitis and was given a course of antibiotics each time, a ritual that began in adolescence and continued through college and into her adult years:

> In retrospect, I think I had asthma. That cough growing up is what an asthmatic cough is to me now, this dry, trying to clear, can't clear, tight feeling. Some quick-acting Ventolin [a brand of albuterol inhaler] and some inhaled steroids will take care of it without antibiotics. I think I'm one of those people that was way over antibiotic'ed because back then, I don't think the medical profession was looking at asthma, particularly in young adults, out of nowhere.

By "out of nowhere," Brenda meant "without a history of allergies." It was not until she was in her late forties, when her cough became persistent, that she was diagnosed with asthma. This cough, Brenda explained, was something that she always experienced following colds; the cough was an acute illness that annually—that is, chronically—appeared in her lungs.

In recent years, medical researchers have paid more and more attention to viruses as asthmatic pathways, in large part in response to the numbers of diagnosed asthma sufferers who identify colds as debilitating triggers for disordered breathing. Indeed, in the NHLBI presentation on phenotypes mentioned above, "infection" is listed as one of the "trigger-induced" phenotypes.[24] But Brenda's teenage experience of what was probably asthma took place before this new medical paradigm had arrived. In other words, there was a moment in asthma's modern history when asthma was understood to be a children's disease, a disease of a particular age group. At that time, doctors were generally not looking for asthma to begin in young adults (at least maybe not in rural New York).[25]

Brenda's age did eventually factor into her asthma diagnosis, albeit later in life. It was during her mandated cardiac stress test at the age of fifty that Brenda's medical team questioned her baseline breathing and registered it as pathological EIA. In this case, it was not her own experience of disordered breathing that signaled anything was amiss. Rather, the parameters established by the performance test marked Brenda's breathing as pathological. Had her breathing not been put under the microscope of a clinical stress test, Brenda may never have named exercise as a context in which she experienced asthma. Like Shaun, Brenda was hesitant to claim her asthma fully, despite having been diagnosed with it twice. "I wouldn't say it impinges on anything," she told me. Many people experience disease as something that presents obstacles to living, and this was not how Brenda thought about her asthma. Nevertheless, when performing against clinical standards, she registered as asthmatic.

Cynthia was another older white woman from a middle-class family in Upstate New York who was diagnosed with asthma later in life:

> I was fifty, and I first noticed it that fall. We had had one of those air inversions that you get in September where it had been really decent fall weather and then all of a sudden this thing comes in and you get this big heavy air mass that comes in and it just presses and it got very, very humid and there was a ton of like, pollen and pollution. And I was out walking, which I should not have been, probably, but I didn't realize I had anything wrong with me. And I had this real reaction, trying to breathe. I didn't think anything of it and it kind of went away, but then I developed a cough and this cough was just—I was coughing all the time. And I was still teaching so I was really trying to control it because I was in the classroom and at night I was hardly sleeping. They tried a variety of different things. You know, well take this medicine and try this medicine and take this thing. And it wasn't getting any better. Then when I was over at the Cape and it was October and it was just so bad, I could not even stay. Can you imagine? I was at the ocean, which you would think it would be cleansing—I couldn't even stay there. I couldn't even sleep at night. I could not sleep. I couldn't even lie down. So we left, Mark and I left after one day and we came home and I called an urgent care and they did this treatment, whatever this is, it's like a breathing treatment. It took a half hour or forty-five minutes and it was almost like I had to continually breathe with this machine and it cleared everything out pretty well. He gave me a prescription for something. They said that they felt that I was going to have to use some kind of maintenance to keep my lungs clear because they thought I had all the symptoms of asthma. I said to them, asthma? I said, we have no asthma in my family. They said, you can develop it.

Cynthia's claim "we have no asthma in my family" speaks to asthma's association with heredity, with family history. This association, built from the dominance of the allergic model of asthma, has been so ingrained in cultural and medical imaginaries that it has taken decades for medical researchers and health care providers to see or think about the disease in any other way. In September 1999, when Cynthia had her first bout with asthma, her doctors looked for other conditions first. Given her age, Cynthia's doctor ran a series of imaging tests to see if her airways were obstructed by tumors. Only after she responded positively to asthma medication—both in the urgent care clinic and later at home—was Cynthia diagnosed with asthma. Cynthia's experience illustrates one of the multiple ways in which an asthma diagnosis can be confirmed: through an assessment of how symptoms and airflow limitation improve once the body receives different kinds of medications.

Diagnostic and treatment standardization is a major and crucial undertaking in the field of asthma research today.[26] As the cases described above illustrate, doctors diagnose and classify asthma in different ways, only some of which breathers recognize as asthma on their own. Of these categories, EIA and allergic asthma are the only two asthma subclasses named by any of the interviewees in my study. In addition to the GINA report mentioned above, NHLBI's National Asthma Education and Prevention Program published a report on diagnostic protocols in 2007 that was the go-to source for asthma management in the United States during the period in which I conducted my research (and it remains a top source). Yet a third document, a 2009 joint statement on "asthma control" by the American Thoracic Society (ATS) and the European Respiratory Society (ERS), recommends that asthma be diagnosed according to how well a patient manages such disease indicators as symptoms, pulmonary function, and use of rescue inhalers and even emergency services.[27] The vast majority of the people I interviewed had received their diagnoses of asthma well before any of these three documents were published. This, too, reflects an element of how asthma is experienced over time: patients continue to experience disease, or the label of disease, even after diagnostic criteria change, but their continuing medical care changes as the medical community revises its standards.

According to the GINA report, an asthma diagnosis can be made after a health care provider identifies characteristic patterns of respiratory symptoms, which could include shortness of breath, chest tightness, coughing, wheezing, and variable expiratory airflow—one dimension of variation in lung function, to be explained in greater detail below. The guidelines list a number of respiratory patterns that likely indicate asthma: if symptoms are worse at night or in the morning; if they are triggered by viral infections, exercise, allergens, changes in weather, laughter, or irritants such as vehicle exhaust, smoke, or strong smells; if there are several different kinds of symptoms; and if symptoms vary over time and in intensity. Variability is a key feature, and one that is increasingly used to diagnose asthma. The GINA report also emphasizes that a patient's evidence of asthma, such as any of the respiratory patterns noted above, should be documented right away, since "the features that are characteristic of asthma may improve spontaneously or with treatment; as a result, it is often more difficult to confirm a diagnosis of asthma once the patient has been started on controller treatment."[28]

The GINA guidelines feature a diagnostic flowchart that walks the doctor through a checklist of sorts, beginning with present respiratory symptoms.[29] If these are typical of asthma, the physician should next explore the patient's individual and family history. This type of information can help the doctor to gauge whether the patient may have had undiagnosed disordered breathing as a child, such as in Brenda's case. Family history is also important because, historically, asthma has seemed to run in families, particularly in the allergic asthma phenotype. Indeed, this was how Cynthia thought about asthma and why she was surprised at her diagnosis— asthma did not run in her family.

If, at this point, all signs point to asthma, then the doctor's next step is to run a pulmonary performance test using a spirometer, a machine that measures the volume and speed of air as it is inhaled and exhaled. For asthma diagnosis and management, the focus is on the exhale. The health care provider first takes a base measure of the patient's forced vital capacity (FVC), which is the amount of air that the patient can forcefully exhale after inhaling as deeply as possible. A related measurement is forced expiratory volume, or the volume of air exhaled, in one second (FEV1). FEV1 and FVC are also measured together, as a ratio. A low FVC level indicates an airway obstruction and possibly airway inflammation—a key indicator of asthma that has been heavily studied. An airflow limitation can signal many different health issues, however, so a low FVC level in itself is not sufficient to diagnose asthma. Instead, the signature airflow limitation associated with asthma is *variability* in lung function, as measured by spirometry. In this context, variability in airflow limitation can be "identified over the course of one day (diurnal variability), from day to day, from visit to visit, or seasonally, or from a reversibility test."[30] "Reversibility" in this context refers to rapid improvement in pulmonary performance after the patient uses medication. There are two distinct scenarios: a bronchodilator is administered in the clinic, and a reversibility test shows marked improvement in peak expiratory flow (PEF) or FEV1 minutes later; or the patient uses a controller medication for several weeks, and pulmonary function is shown to improve from daily medication use.

The spirometer is not the only tool used to measure and assess lung function in people with asthma. The peak flow meter, a very different kind of pulmonary performance technology, is used to measure how fast an individual can exhale, or peak expiratory flow. In contrast with the spirometer, the peak flow meter is a simple, handheld device. Styles vary, but the typical meter displays a numeric and color-coded scale along its side so that the user can easily see the results and keep track of differences in how well he or she exhales from day to day or even from morning to night. The higher the score, the less obstructed the airways. Peak flow meters are a low-cost, personal technology that health care providers prescribe for patients to use as part of their daily disease management. As personal disease management tools, peak flow meters provide information that is neither as robust nor as reliable as that produced by spirometers, according to clinical standards. In fact, the GINA guidelines emphasize that a patient tracking PEF should use the same peak flow meter each time, since measurements may differ up to 20 percent from meter to meter.[31] Particularly when used by trained operators, well-maintained spirometers are more accurate.[32] Nevertheless, because of their low cost and ease of use, peak flow meters are more accessible tools for asthma care. Peak flow meters can help asthma patients build knowledge about their illness in ways that spirometers cannot. The value of PEF tests grows over time, as the patient takes measurements day after day, week after week. The utility of a PEF reading, in other words, depends on the patient's establishment of baseline pulmonary functions, so that readings below the baseline can reliably be understood to signal when there might be underlying inflammation or other forms of obstruction limiting expiratory airflow. Variation can be assessed only if there is a clear baseline against which subsequent readings can be judged. The successful use of a peak flow meter thus depends on proper and regular use by the asthma sufferer.

Despite the emphasis on measuring airflow limitation in the asthma management literature, my impression based on fieldwork is that pulmonary performance is largely absent from disease management in practice. In eight years, I did not meet a single asthma sufferer who used a peak flow meter as part of a care regimen. Some reported using peak flow meters when first diagnosed, often in childhood, but they had not sustained this practice. When asked why this was so, my interviewees offered several explanations, but they frequently returned to their preference for understanding their disease from within their own care regimens and experiences. Kevin, for example, never found value in pulmonary performance tests:

> When you have your physicals they always do spirometry or if I go in
> and I'm complaining of a bronchial infection, they do a peak flow
> meter. But the strange thing is that the standards that they set for that
> are sort of—I think that there has not been a lot of science done around
> different bodies and how the peak flow reading works. Because I mean,
> they look at a chart and they say, oh, this is your weight and this is
> your height and this is your age. So your peak flow should be X. Every
> time, every single time I have ever used the peak flow meter I am above
> and beyond the top of the chart. Even when I'm sick, I'm way above

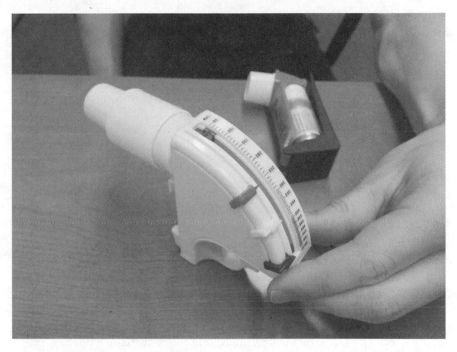

An asthma sufferer holds a peak flow meter. A rescue inhaler is on the table behind it. Photograph by Alison Kenner.

and beyond the chart. Frankly, based on my experiences, I think it's sort of a bullshit measure.

This was a complaint I heard frequently: peak flow meters do not provide any useful information. At the same time, however, it was clear that many of my interviewees did not understand what information the readings were meant to relay about the disease—namely, that variations in peak flow readings could indicate airway obstruction and underlying inflammation that could make them more susceptible to attacks. The lack of understanding of this purpose among those interviewed says as much about patient education as it does about the peak flow meter's actual utility in disease management. Most of the people I interviewed, however, had been diagnosed more than five years before, and many had been diagnosed decades previously, during childhood. In cases where the asthma diagnosis was made during childhood, interviewees often told me that care instructions and disease information had been directed to their parents. It seems as though their health care providers did not always review instructions for peak flow meter use, either with the patients or with their parents.

When I asked Kevin if he thought regular use of a peak flow meter in daily care practices could increase the utility of the pulmonary function tests performed in the clinic by establishing a target value for the individual, he agreed that it might. If he "did it for a long period of time and actually got a baseline," he said, he might see fluctuations that paralleled his symptoms and the seasons when he experienced them. But he also made clear that consistent, daily monitoring would be the only way to make this measurement useful. Assessed against "objective" numbers, he asserted, the readings would be meaningless.

Part of what I found interesting about this conversation was that Kevin was among the most "adherent" asthmatics I interviewed over the years — meaning that he diligently used his controller medication twice a day. He had a daily care regimen already, so why not simply add in a peak flow reading? It only takes a minute. Kevin told me that implementing a daily peak flow reading did not seem worth the effort, particularly since he had already figured out on his own what the peak flow meter was designed to tell him: "The reality is that I physically know when I'm not breathing right. I don't need an instrument to tell me what I already know." This stance, that the asthma sufferer recognizes the signs of illness better than clinicians can or than biomedical readings can reveal, was repeated across a number of interviews. I will return to it in the next chapter, but here the point I want to make is that this belief in personal expertise was strongly associated with higher degrees of disease severity and long duration of illness. Those interviewees who had mild or intermittent asthma or had lived with disordered breathing for only a few years had less confidence in their knowledge of their asthma.

Patients' perceptions of disordered breathing may differ from what is considered clinically acceptable, as happened in Brenda's case.[33] Diagnostic standards may have changed, but Brenda has always lived her life a certain way; for her, something that registers as compromised respiratory function on a spirometer does not feel like an impingement on her quality of life. Whether she knew it or not, asthma is something she has lived with for nearly forty years. Like Shaun, Brenda does not see herself as a chronic asthmatic because her symptoms are, *by her definition,* episodic, occurring only once or twice a year with viruses. Brenda therefore uses medication only rarely. Although she has a prescription for a rescue inhaler, she noted that she rarely has to use it, "with the very mild asthma that I have."

Outgrowing Disease

Sam coughed for the third time in ten minutes. It was not a significant, body-wrenching cough, but rather a mild nuance. A thirty-one-year-old white Tennessean from a working-class family, Sam "grew out of" asthma after high school. He told me that he has been symptom-free since age eighteen or nineteen. His seasonal allergies went away a few years ago too, in his late twenties, so he no longer needed monthly allergy shots. An out-of-state move, he told me, forever rid him of his seasonal burden.

Asthmatics have described this sort of waxing and waning of allergies on countless occasions. These stories typically feature a move, either to a new building or to a new ecosystem. New contexts speak to our bodies differently than the ones in which we have history. Life-story plot changes make all the difference for illness experiences, and such embodied twists can alter the tempo and direction of a person's asthma narrative. Although science struggles to document how temporal and spatial changes in asthma reflect biological change, common knowledge suggests that allergies can change over time and place.[34] The idea that a person can "grow out of" asthma came up repeatedly in my interviews. For every asthmatic I interviewed, I have met two more who told me they grew out of the disease. Asthma is merely a childhood memory to them. Interviews and anecdotes suggest that many doctors support the idea that children can grow out of asthma, just as they can grow out of training wheels, dental retainers, and other temporary aids. This notion perhaps also reflects earlier cultural beliefs about asthma as a form of childhood anxiety and psychosomatic stress.[35]

In contrast to these narratives, a number of medical studies have shown that most people do not "outgrow" asthma. Asthma that was active in childhood may become dormant in teenagers and young adults, but it often reemerges later in life, in different ways.[36] Vic was a thirty-two-year-old allergic asthmatic whose parents had migrated from India to Upstate New York before he was born. He was diagnosed with asthma in the first grade and lived for the next decade with a severe form of the disease. There was a brief stretch of time after that when he believed he had outgrown it, but then it returned, in all its severity:

> There was a recurrence. For a long time I sort of told myself that I was going to outgrow it and then as I entered sort of my late teens, it felt like things were getting better and there was a theory where I was able to work out more, I was able to go outside and do things more and I felt like, hey, maybe I'm outgrowing this thing. But then it came back and I think at that point in time I thought, well maybe I'm not going to outgrow it. And maybe I need to come up with different ways of dealing with this for the rest of my life and it's not just like a childhood problem that is going to go away later.

Time comes into the asthmatic condition in many ways. Asthma is anything but linear. Vic named his experience with asthma as a recurrence—

something that was there, then gone, and then back again, but different. His story is fairly typical, in that many adults with asthma may have experienced it as a different condition in childhood, one that was more or less severe, with different triggers and sensations. To recognize the similarities in these differences, asthmatics need somatic sense and perception (attunement); they also need to be open to the possibility of recurrence.

When people with asthma mention outgrowing the disease, they are often referring to differences in severity, such as the frequency, intensity, or quantity of symptoms. For physicians, however, "severity" is a measurable, clinical factor. Clinical severity includes the breather's illness experience but also includes the amount of medication needed to control symptoms. The level of asthma control is defined by "the extent to which the manifestations of asthma can be observed in the patient, or have been reduced or removed by treatment."[37] Doctors assess asthma severity by scoring whether a patient has experienced any of the following four disease dimensions in the past month: daytime asthma symptoms more than twice a week, waking up in the night with symptoms, needing a rescue inhaler more than twice a week, and limiting activities because of asthma. The patient's asthma is considered to be well controlled if the patient has not experienced any of these four criteria in the past month. If the patient has experienced one or two of these criteria, the asthma is considered to be partly controlled. If the patient meets three or four of the criteria, the asthma is considered to be uncontrolled. Doctors prescribe medication types and levels based on the patient's level of asthma control.

The three degrees of asthma severity—mild, moderate, and severe—map on to these definitions of control. *Mild asthma* is the term applied to cases that are well controlled with a SABA drug as needed; in some cases, a patient who also requires a low dose of an inhaled corticosteroid (ICS) may be considered to have mild asthma. Inhaled corticosteroids are the most common form of controller medication; doses are taken daily, in the morning and/or at night. *Moderate asthma* refers to cases that require a controller medication, such as an ICS or a long-acting beta-2 agonist, to keep the disease under control; a patient with moderate asthma also uses a SABA inhaler as needed, when symptoms arise. The final category, *severe asthma,* comprises those cases that require moderate to high doses of controller medications to keep symptoms controlled. In some cases, patients with severe asthma may also require other medications to treat comorbidities that are a factor in the disease. No matter the degree of severity, asthma control must be monitored constantly, so that the treatment regimen—and, specifically, amounts of medication—can be adjusted for the current state of disease. This is often referred to as the stepwise approach.

As the guidelines in the GINA report suggest, breathers who have lived with the disease for most of their lives often report distinct illness cycles. Their asthma may become uncontrolled for a number of reasons. They might have a difficult year, sometimes marked by a cold or virus that lasts all winter, or perhaps they experience changes in environment or lifestyle. Sometimes asthma control varies in relation to the seasons. Lisa, a white, middle-class college student in her early twenties, noted how different seasons correlate with differences in air quality and her symptoms:

> It's different, like in the summer, the humidity, you can feel the tightness and stuff, but in the winter is when I have the shortness of breath. It's just terrible in the wintertime. A few years ago, I was using my inhaler every once in a while, but then in the wintertime I was using it every four hours. The most I could use it. And I still wasn't really getting relief from it. It was pretty bad in the wintertime. And I wouldn't ever get the relief from the inhaler. So I felt like for months I had shortness of breath. That's when I finally went to the specialist.

Lisa was one of a few people I interviewed who had been diagnosed with asthma as an infant. During childhood, she received nebulizer treatments regularly, but it was not until winter during her first year of high school that her asthma became uncontrolled. During that time, she felt as though she was out of breath for months, despite using her rescue inhaler several times a day. It was only after Lisa went to an asthma specialist and was put on a daily controller medication that her asthma was brought under control. Since then, Lisa has been using an ICS. She said that she did not like it, but it was a trade-off she was willing to make in order to breathe more easily. Since high school, Lisa has had a moderate form of asthma that has been, for the most part, well controlled.

Amelia, a white, nineteen-year-old college student from a middle-class family, had lived her entire life in rural Upstate New York. Like Lisa, she was born with asthma and had been diagnosed with it around the age of one. Amelia and her parents thought she had grown out of the disease—a pattern documented when asthma develops in children under the age of five—but it returned after a long dormancy:[38]

> I semi grew out of it a little bit. I didn't have any attacks from when I was probably around six up until eighth grade, and then I had pneumonia and then I got it back. Then every time I had a cold, I would get it back. And when I was running. I had very bad asthma attacks whenever I ran. And then whenever the weather changed or I got a cold it came back.

Pneumonia reignited Amelia's dormant asthma, which she began experiencing in a number of contexts. Her symptom pattern, however, stayed consistent: "Wheezing—always started it. That is how I knew an asthma attack was coming on." Colds and changes in the weather were the most common triggers for Amelia. When I asked her how often she used her rescue inhaler, she said whenever she needed it: "The time when the seasons are changing or something, I would have to take it every certain number of hours. And it would have to be pretty regular. But other than that, I would just have it with me." Things had changed since she moved to college, however:

> It's not the way it was when I got it back in eighth grade, that was
> pretty severe. I don't need to carry an inhaler around with me at all
> times. I usually do anyway, just in case. But it's not like if the seasons
> change—that used to happen to me when it got colder or when it got
> warmer, I used to need my inhaler. But I don't know, I don't really think
> I would consider myself an asthmatic anymore.

Amelia's voice revealed her uncertainty about how she would be categorized today. I asked her when she had last used her rescue inhaler, and she told me it was back in the fall, when she got a cold. Viruses still triggered a mild version of asthma for her. Even at the height of her illness, however, in 2004 and 2005, Amelia had never been prescribed an ICS.

If asthma is heterogeneous and multiple in its symptoms, temporality, and environmental and behavioral triggers, then asthmatics' experiences, perceptions, and responses to their disease are equally multiple and varied. Beliefs about disease state and treatment ranged widely among those I interviewed. Some felt that disordered breathing was not a problem worthy of diagnosis and treatment; others, like Cynthia, simply did not want to "mess around" with the effects of asthma, even in its dormant phases:

> I was a little hesitant. Because if you think about it, if you stop and
> think about everything you do in a day—especially if you are an active
> person, if you feel that there is something that is going to—if you are
> afraid, something in your body is making you afraid to do things, then
> that really is a quality of life issue. So if you are treated or you know
> you are getting treatment—there is something about knowing—being
> proactive and saying, I need to get to the bottom of this. It affects your
> life and when you get to be my age, you don't want to be messing
> around with that kind of stuff.

Given the fluctuations—the periodicity—of asthma, health care providers generally administer treatment through step-up and step-down approaches.

Cynthia's doctor, for example, had wanted to step down her daily controller medication dose from morning and evening to just once a day. Those breathers I interviewed who were resistant to using pharmaceuticals still recognized the value of drugs when their symptoms emerged. As one man in his mid-forties told me, "There is nothing worse than not being able to fucking breathe."

For people who no longer experience asthma, however, having the diagnosis follow them around, even after it seems irrelevant, can be an annoyance. Tyler, a white, twenty-nine-year-old middle-class man from Albany, New York, found that his teenage diagnosis remained relevant, in his doctors' minds, long after he felt his symptoms had disappeared:

> They diagnosed me with asthma when I was in high school—oddly
> enough, even now they still like to diagnose me with that even though
> I haven't had a problem with asthma in years. Anytime I go in for any
> type of ailment, they will be like, oh are you still on your inhalers? And
> I will say no, I went off of them. And they are like, oh you should go
> back on them. Which is getting kind of annoying, because I don't need
> it. I haven't been on it for more than five years and if I go in with a
> common cold, I don't want them to tell me its asthma related.

Whereas some people, like Amelia, Sam, and Tyler, felt they had outgrown their asthma, others just thought it was better managed and controlled than when they were younger. Kevin, for example, described his asthma as "less intense" in his thirties than it was when he was younger. He attributed this to his own embodied knowledge and care practices, which had enabled him to become more efficient at controlling his disease:

> I don't believe that people grow out of asthma. I think it's a myth. I
> think what it comes down to is that people become more aware of their
> triggers and they become more aware of what environmental hazards
> there are. So they just are less likely to be bothered by it, because they
> just figured out what it is that causes their asthma.

Like many children and teens with asthma, Kevin had been told by doctors, his parents, and other caregivers that he would likely outgrow the disease after adolescence. This never came to pass. Kevin expressed the idea that the myth of outgrowing asthma renders patient knowledge and care invisible. This knowledge accrues with experience, but it is experience anchored in asthmatic attunement to changing timescapes. As he told me, "I don't think we realize how sensitive we are to our environment until we remove ourselves from those places and then go back into them and realize exactly how intense that can be. We become normalized."

In this chapter I have described the many names and various labels that patients and medical professionals use to talk about asthma, but the disease can also be something that people have no language for. Asthma is an illness that can be too ephemeral to talk about; in other cases, its presence may simply be assumed. Either way, asthma often goes undiscussed. In an exchange I had with Geoff, a white, thirty-six-year-old working-class man from Philadelphia, he marveled as I named and described the different kinds of asthma. "I had no idea asthma was so complicated," he told me, noting that his asthma is singular—meaning that he has only one kind of asthma. He was diagnosed as an allergic asthmatic during childhood. Yet as Geoff and I talked, he recounted many different conditions and objects that trigger his asthma, including everything from cold air to cats. Like other asthma sufferers I interviewed, Geoff described how the disease strains his relationships in different ways—it limits his ability to engage in outdoor activities such as biking and skiing, and it prevents him from living with cats or dogs, a reality that eventually ended a relationship with a longtime partner.

I was struck when Geoff thanked me for doing this work, for giving asthma a language: "I never know how to describe it to people so I feel like the people around me never really know what it's like. I had no idea that there was a language for talking about asthma. I wish I had known how to communicate like this with people." In some ways, asthma is common; it is an old enough disease that it is often taken for granted, on multiple levels. Asthma's age and history, however, have shaped our knowledge of the disease in ways that make it difficult for us to identify and name asthma today. Some of the people I spoke with, like Shaun, felt that their disease experience lacked coherence, and they wanted to make sense of it. Others wanted more information than their doctors had given them. They felt that the information their doctors provided was incomplete—although this is arguably a sentiment shared by a majority of Americans regarding their interactions with medical professionals. While they could, of course, turn to the internet, online searches do not help to clarify the ambiguity, the variability, or, more important, the lived experience of asthma.

Those I interviewed usually asked me what causes asthma. I responded by pointing them to professional associations and patient organizations, and, on some occasions, to the scientific literature. Often I turned the discussion around, asking them more questions in the hope that our dialogue over their disease narratives might reveal some insight into their conditions. The truth was that many of their questions have yet to be answered by the asthma research community. The diagnosed asthma sufferers I interviewed are experts on their own disordered breathing, but not always experts on the disease recognized as asthma. Many of the asthmatics I spoke with, like Shaun, felt that *asthma,* the disease, did not match their experience. Some denied having "real" asthma, or reported that they had grown out of the disease. Although they did not consider themselves patients with a disease, they were experts on breathing, atmosphere, and environmental exposure.[39]

Asthma's multiplicity has a variety of effects. For people living with asthma, waning or changing symptoms may lead them to believe that they have outgrown the disease, a viewpoint that their doctors or caregivers sometimes echo. That individuals may experience the disease differently over time can lead to complications in their treatment, and especially to nonadherence to medication regimens. Although his doctors suggested he might grow out of the disease, Tim Brookes was one of the unlucky asthmatics who did not. He just became better attuned to the multiple forms of his breathing problems, which ultimately included life-threatening attacks more severe than any he had experienced during childhood. For others, like Cynthia and Kevin, asthma triggers and symptoms remain stable over most of the life course; this may help to explain why so many asthmatics, like Sam, stop experiencing major attacks, stop seeking asthma treatment and taking medications, and sometimes even stop thinking they have a disease condition. As Brookes's and Kevin's accounts suggest, disordered breathing becomes part of normal life rather than something that would drive a person to seek treatment. Brookes notes, "This is the paradox of chronic illness: the patient grows around the disease, like an oak tree engulfing a barbed-wire fence."[40]

Asthma's multiplicity has also been a problem for researchers working to understand causation and molecular mechanisms and, of course, to develop targeted drugs. That asthma looks different and is experienced differently from one person to the next, and even within the same person over time, frustrates biomedical paradigms designed for comparability across subjects. This can present problems not only for asthma patients but also for doctors treating such patients and scientists researching the disease. Targeted drug treatments cannot be developed and tested without precise pathophysiological classification. Scientific publications and research programs reference asthma phenotypes with increasing regularity, but these distinctions have not yet produced targeted treatment regimens; researchers have not yet settled on a list of phenotypes, and it is unclear what phenotype differentiation will mean for patient care. So far, there are no drug recommendations for specific phenotypes.[41] Instead, doctors and patients manage asthma according to classic patterns, of which atopic and exercise-induced asthma are the most common. Treatments look the same as they did ten or fifteen years ago, when long-term "controller" or "maintenance" medications first hit the market. These medications do just that: they work to control the risk of a variable, complex environmental health epidemic by maintaining functional breathing among those affected. In my research, however, I often saw a significant disconnect between patient knowledge and care and biomedical knowledge and management regimens.

Asthma's heterogeneous, multiple, and variable dynamics mean that those with the condition experience a wide range of perceptions and care responses; these perceptions and responses can change over time as the disease changes. Like Brookes, many asthmatics experience several types of asthma. Most asthmatics describe these various types as distinctly different from one another. Sometimes their descriptions resemble and overlap with the descriptions of phenotype groups in the scientific literature, and sometimes they do not. Like biomedical researchers who feel the inadequacy of such a general term as *asthma,* asthmatics know that their disordered breathing is multiple. While both asthmatics and researchers are able to classify the multiple forms of asthma by emplacing disordered breathing in timescapes that trigger symptoms, the processes and tools used by the two groups are distinct. Clinical practices are organized around a standardized language that enables diagnosis, assessment, and treatment, but these practices still depend on the emplaced knowledge that asthma sufferers cultivate through attunement. Indeed, clinical understanding of asthma phenotypes is based in the narratives of breathers' emplaced experiences. There are no tests that will produce a number that tells whether an individual has asthma or not.

These illness dimensions matter not only for how asthma is known, for people with disordered breathing and those who treat and study it, but also for asthma care—how asthmatics, their doctors, researchers, and public health workers think the disease should be treated.

CHAPTER TWO

Three Modes of Control
as Asthma Care

> Respiratory rhythm is a function of our awareness of our situation in
> the world.
> — Georges Canguilhem, *On the Normal and the Pathological*

Asthmatics respond to their disordered breathing in different ways, some
of which their care providers might not recommend. Their responses
are anchored in asthmatic attunement, a feeling for disordered breathing
as it emerges. Attention to specific sensation and force is a key dimension
of asthma sufferers' awareness of symptoms, but *where* they are at the
moment of attack matters for care, too. How a person responds in the
moment of disordered breathing conveys much about the individual's disease, of course, but it also reveals how that person practices care while
emplaced in a layered, entangled world. Economic decisions, ideas about
immunity and resilience, relationships with animals, physical safety, and
the grateful-hateful stance that many people have toward pharmaceuticals
all factor into response-in-the-moment. The way an asthma sufferer relates
to these things is more often than not framed by the time and place of
breath—in the body and in the world. Yet asthma is more than just disordered breathing in the moment. Asthma is chronic if episodic; it can be
rendered invisible over time, and increasingly it is defined by biological
characteristics that exceed the symptoms through which breathers know
their disease.

Mark, born and raised in Upstate New York, was thirty-five when we
sat down to do our interview. I met Mark through our mutual professional networks, and the interview was conducted in Southern California,
where we were both attending a conference. Neither of us lived in Southern California at the time of the interview, so our conversation included
commentary on the region's atmosphere, as well as the air quality in the
conference venue itself. An academic who had moved frequently for school,
fieldwork, and jobs, Mark offered a narrative of his asthmatic experiences
that was peppered with accounts of environmental encounters that had

triggered life-threatening attacks. He had been diagnosed with allergic asthma at the age of six and had lived with the disease in its severe form for most of his life. The way that Mark and many other interviewees talked about their relationships to medication reflects a dominant orientation toward pharmaceuticals in the United States today—that of a fear of biochemical dependence. Mark described how he measures his use of a rescue inhaler according to the kind of asthma attack he is having and the conditions in which the attack occurs:

> When I was younger, it was the feeling of wheezing—like if I felt it in my throat or if I felt it in my lungs, I would immediately turn to my rescue inhaler. As I have gotten older, I don't want to use the medication as much, so I will still feel the sort of tingling in my throat or in my lungs or something but often I try to slow down and control my breathing and sort of calm down, rather than turning to the rescue inhaler immediately. If it feels itchy inside, to me I know that I need my medication. So I do get acute asthma attacks where it's hard for me to tell how much longer I can go on breathing. That has happened in my adult life as well. So I know what that feels like and I have had serious asthma attacks as an adult where I have to get ambulatory care or something. And so from my perspective, there is a point at which I just don't feel like remaining calm and breathing slowly or even taking my rescue inhaler is going to work.

Mark thus viewed some of his asthma attacks as allowing for a range of possible responses, while other kinds prompted him to use a rescue inhaler immediately.

As Mark noted, he found that he wanted to use medication less as he got older, and instead began trying to exert embodied control when symptoms arose. "The way that I think about breathing has changed over time," he told me, emphasizing that he had tried to make himself stronger and more resilient, too:

> I took so many inhalers as a child. But I started weaning myself off of that, I started doing more exercise. I tried to build up my fitness, because I didn't want to take the steroids all the time. There are a lot of side effects to taking those things. So I developed this regime. But then I was told no. Like you really should be taking the steroids because that is a better allocation of resources than if you get sick and then we need to hospitalize you.

Mark's health care provider was not wrong: taking an inhaled corticosteroid and/or other kinds of daily controller medications is much more cost-effective than using emergency services or being hospitalized as the result of an attack, both things that Mark had needed to do as an adult. This economic trade-off between controller medication use and hospitalization has been cited widely in public health communications about asthma, from governmental and nongovernmental organizations alike. The message is that asthmatics' resistance to using controller medications raises costs for U.S. taxpayers. Thus, doctors, public health workers, and advocacy organizations exert tremendous effort to encourage people with diagnosed asthma to take controller medications, particularly if their asthma is not well controlled or if they have a moderate or severe form of the disease.[1]

The asthma sufferers I spoke with displayed a mix of ambivalence and hostility toward pharmaceuticals, and especially toward controller medications. Of those who used controller medications, many acknowledged that they needed the drugs to breathe, and so took them despite the possibility of unknown long-term side effects. Without controller medications, their daily lives might be unbearable, unbreathable. Others expressed frustration and outright hostility toward the pharmaceutical industry. Among all the asthmatics I interviewed, Tyler voiced the most extreme views on this subject:

> I personally believe that the medication that gets prescribed in this country is only there to keep you alive long enough to make more money off of you, more prescriptions. So I think that they are ultimately doing more harm than good. So if you can get through—if you can do other things, whether it be exercising, being healthy, or just kind of doing a whole immunity type thing where you are giving yourself small doses of the thing you're sensitive to, I think you are better off in the long term to not be addicted. That is ultimately what it is. I think there are so many people that are addicted to medications. Even if they are doing something good for you, it's doing something else that is bad. Anytime you watch a commercial for a drug, there is a laundry list of things that are bad for you. So I don't know offhand, like off the top of my head, what those bad side effects are for asthma, but the one thing that—the only thing I can think of is the one time you don't have your inhaler, because you left it at your friend's house or you left it in the car or the plane lost your luggage and now you need it, and now you are going to die because you need that medication. I don't want to have that situation where I have to have something, and if I don't, it's going to cause harm to me.

Aside from his perspective on the pharmaceutical industry—which might be characterized as cynical or suspicious—Tyler expressed two other dynamics that are the focus of this chapter. The first is the idea that an individual can develop nonpharmaceutical strategies to "get through" asthma symptoms. The second is the idea that medication cultivates biochemical dependence and thus dependence on an industry: the asthma sufferer must be on drugs for life in order to breathe.[2]

In this chapter I explore these dynamics by focusing on the practices that breathers use to care for themselves. These care practices display asthmatics' close attention not only to what is happening within their bodies in relation to the surrounding world (attunement) but also to the larger social and material conditions that shape their experience (emplacement). There are important temporal and affective differences between attunement and emplacement, which I will explain in my discussion of the narratives to come. My second aim in this chapter is to show how asthmatic attunement and emplaced care contrast with the discourse of *asthma control* that has become a cornerstone of treatment guidelines and public health recommendations in clinical arenas. While those who prescribe controller medications attempt to minimize future risk, asthma sufferers talk about breath control in the present, as Mark conveyed. This brings me to the chapter's third argument: that asthma sufferers and those who treat asthma approach the problem of *control* through different timescapes. Understanding care in asthma requires paying attention to shifts in temporality, whether that means controlling symptoms over a four-week span, controlling for future risk of adverse outcomes, or controlling the breath from inhale to exhale.

Future Risk in Control Cultures

While the medical literature has referred to something called "asthma control" since at least the mid-twentieth century, it is only in the past decade that asthma experts have offered an explicit definition of this term. A clear definition allows doctors and researchers to operationalize the concept. According to the guidelines in the 2018 report of the Global Initiative for Asthma (discussed in chapter 1), doctors should assess asthma control at the time of diagnosis as well as in all subsequent visits, or, as the report puts it, "at every opportunity." The report states that asthma control represents control over symptoms as well as over "future risk of adverse outcomes":

> The level of asthma control is the extent to which the manifestations of
> asthma can be observed in the patient, or have been reduced or
> removed by treatment. It is determined by the interaction between the
> patient's genetic background, underlying disease processes, the

treatment that they are taking, environment, and psychosocial factors.

Asthma control has two domains: symptom control (previously called "current clinical control") and future risk of adverse outcomes. Both should always be assessed. Lung function is an important part of the assessment of future risk; it should be measured at the start of treatment, after 3–6 months of treatment (to identify the patient's personal best), and periodically thereafter for ongoing risk assessment.[3]

As noted in chapter 1, medical professionals consider change in lung function over time, measured through the use of either a peak flow meter or a spirometer, to be the gold standard for determining a patient's level of asthma control. Four weeks is the key time span used in the clinical assessment of asthma control. Doctors ask about daytime and nighttime asthma attacks, symptom frequency and severity, how often the patient's activities are limited by asthma, and—assuming the person has a prior diagnosis—how often the patient has used a rescue inhaler in the past month. GINA recommends that physicians use a numerical asthma control questionnaire, which may help to cut down on the ambiguity that might otherwise characterize the way patients reflect on how their disease is affecting them. For patients with a prior diagnosis, this assessment is meant to investigate adherence and evaluate how well prescribed medications are working, or if the disease condition has changed—as it so often does with asthma. Recall that Cynthia had been instructed to step down her use of her controller medication, from twice a day to once (see chapter 1). Her doctor made this recommendation only after establishing that Cynthia's symptoms had been well controlled for a number of years and that her lung function had been steady.

"Future risk of adverse outcomes" is a relatively new category of concern in asthma treatment, appearing in professional association and public health publications of the asthma research community only in the past decade. The GINA report defines adverse outcomes as "exacerbations, fixed airflow limitation, and side effects of medications."[4] The risk of future exacerbations is the most prominent among the listed risk outcomes.[5] Exacerbations, or flare-ups, include the iconic asthma attack—a symptom event where the person cannot breathe—but the term also refers to a broader spectrum of illness indicators. An exacerbation might take the form of a gradual worsening of disordered breathing over the course of a week or a month; a person does not necessarily need to have had an asthma attack to have experienced an exacerbation. Perhaps the breather develops a cough, or has more breathlessness or chest tightness, but these symptoms never progress into an attack. So, whereas an attack is a single, severe event, an exacerbation of asthma can entail a wider duration and greater range of symptoms. The concept of exacerbations gets at the low-grade chronicity of disordered breathing, which can affect quality of life in many different ways. The GINA report states, however, that symptoms themselves, "although an important outcome for patients, and themselves a strong predictor of future risk of exacerbations, are not sufficient on their own for assessing asthma."[6]

The report details a number of reasons health care providers should be skeptical of relying solely on patients' visible, felt symptoms of disease. First, the appearance of "controlled" asthma might mask underlying airway inflammation. Although it is unclear what the long-term outcomes of chronic airway inflammation are—airway remodeling and lowered lung function are the two most discussed—health care professionals want to guard against such inflammation. Second, respiratory symptoms may be brought on by other conditions, such as comorbidities or a "lack of fitness." In other words, even when patients have symptom control, continual assessment is needed to make sure that no underlying conditions are contributing to respiratory disorder. Third, mental health conditions may affect how patients experience and report symptoms. Finally, some patients have low lung function, but without telltale respiratory symptoms. This seems to be more common in some asthma phenotypes than in others.[7] While a decline in lung function with aging is normal in healthy adults, asthma sufferers may have an accelerated decline if, for example, they are not taking appropriate medications.

Given this framing by the GINA report, *anyone* diagnosed with asthma appears to be at risk of future adverse outcomes. The document provides two examples of asthma control. In the first, the patient's asthma is well controlled; in the second, the asthma is poorly controlled:

> Ms X has good asthma symptom control, but she is at increased risk of future exacerbations because she has had a severe exacerbation within the last year.
>
> Mr Y has poor asthma symptom control. He also has several additional risk factors for future exacerbations including low lung function, current smoking, and poor medication adherence.[8]

Although Ms. X has good asthma control in the moment—and is likely an adherent patient—both she and Mr. Y are at risk of future exacerbations. The definition of being at risk of future adverse outcomes seems to encompass everyone. Who is not at risk?[9]

The 2009 joint statement by the American Thoracic Society and the European Respiratory Society, published nearly a decade before the GINA report, describes future risks for asthma similarly, as "loss of control in the near or distant future, exacerbations, accelerated decline in lung function, and treatment-related side effects."[10] But the ATS/ERS statement also refers to financial or economic risks, such as unscheduled use of health care services and missed work. Indeed, within U.S. public health arenas, the asthma epidemic has more often than not been framed as an issue affecting the national economy. Many publications open with descriptions of the nation's economic "asthma burden," which some reports place as high as $81 billion a year from hospitalizations, use of emergency services, and lost wages.[11] These costs stem largely from "uncontrolled" asthma, which occurs when the disease is untreated or undertreated.

In 1989, on the heels of the emergence of the U.S. asthma epidemic, the National Heart, Lung, and Blood Institute established the National Asthma Education and Prevention Program (NAEPP) to raise awareness about asthma as a disease among multiple constituency groups. The NAEPP's mission was, in part, to coordinate activities across federal agencies, but also to support "effective control of asthma by encouraging a partnership among Federal agencies, patients, physicians, and other health professionals through modern treatment and education programs."[12] In 2008, the NAEPP established the National Asthma Control Initiative (NACI), whose overarching focus is to circulate and reinforce the clinical protocols laid out in the NAEPP's 2007 guidelines for the diagnosis and management of asthma.[13] NACI boils the guidelines down to the following six evidence-based action items for asthma sufferers and their health care providers, with the overarching goal of "improv[ing] asthma control and transform[ing] the lives of people with asthma": use inhaled corticosteroids; use written asthma action plans to guide patient self-management; assess asthma severity at the initial visit; assess and monitor asthma control and adjust treatment if needed; schedule follow-up visits at periodic intervals; and control environmental exposures that worsen the patient's asthma.[14] These are the pillars of asthma care, understood as necessary to control not only asthma symptoms but also future risk.

NACI's mission is broad, targeting multiple stakeholders in the arena of asthma care: health care professionals, including doctors and clinics; patients and their caregivers; and schools and other providers of child care. But NACI's message also reaches out beyond these three classic audiences to others affected by asthma's financial impacts, including states, communities, and government–community coalitions; employers, employees, and work sites; and public and private insurers.[15] In this configuration, everyone is implicated in and responsible for asthma control. Nevertheless, the six action items concentrate on what individual asthmatics and their providers need to do. The first five items focus on what happens in the clinical context. Only the last item, concerning the reduction of environmental exposures, points to a broader context, and even here, the action remains focused on what individuals can do in their personal, everyday lives, rather than at the level of the public or collective space. The lack of public health–oriented language on the environment is striking in a statement that begins by invoking the public cost of the asthma epidemic and assigns responsibility for reducing that cost to everyone.

As Joseph Dumit has shown, the idea of future risk and the way it has been mobilized in clinical arenas means that everyone in the United States is a candidate for treatments with prescription medicines, even in the absence of symptoms.[16] In the same way that arbitrary numbers developed through mass clinical trials set the benchmarks for risk categories in heart disease and cholesterol analysis, lung function tests operate to define disease for breathers, even when they feel their disease is controlled and not limiting their lives in any way. The work of NACI puts future risk on the national agenda; as a public communication program, NACI works to ensure that all stakeholders understand that asthma control is about future risk. Health care professionals need to follow and advocate for the above framework—instructing patients to take daily medications to keep inflammation and airway responsiveness controlled, measuring and reporting lung function, assessing quality of life and patient perceptions of disease, and performing regular checkups—to help protect patients from the future risks of asthma, which may include symptoms, decreased lung function, and medication side effects. Everyone is responsible for making sure that patients succeed in these treatment practices.[17] These definitions of control, however, contrast sharply with the ways asthma sufferers describe and experience control in the context of disordered breathing.

A Different Kind of Disease Control

> Sometimes they want to put me on that twice a day and I'm always like, I'm gonna use it twice a day? My asthma is controlled normally when I'm healthy. So that's been kind of frustrating because I hear it all the time. Even the doctor I have been going to my entire life, he said, you should do this. And it's just like, I have my asthma under control, I don't want a medication for it. I know how to deal with it. It's my asthma, I get it.

Greg is a twenty-eight-year-old white, middle-class man from a small New England town. Like Amelia and Lisa, discussed in chapter 1, he was diagnosed with asthma as an infant. His early childhood wheezing developed into allergic asthma, and ever since, Greg has had breathing difficulty in a range of contexts—during exercise, in the presence of mold and cats, and when he gets sick, which is what he was referring to in saying that his asthma is controlled when he is healthy. The only time he really felt like he needed extra assistance from a daily medication was when he was getting over a virus and his breathing was disordered. Otherwise, Greg felt confident in caring for his asthma on his own, without a controller medication. He had no problem using his rescue inhaler as needed. But it was also clear that Greg did not always carry his inhaler with him. He described many times during which he coped with disordered breathing without his inhaler.

When Greg spoke of "control," he was referring to something very different from the kind of control that asthma researchers describe. When I asked him how he *feels* his asthma, he provided a nuanced articulation of asthmatic attunement:

> It's like, it's not a shortness of breath but it's like, the breaths are not as full. For me, it's very obvious at this point. Then, if I'm in the middle of something, if I know that I need to complete this task and I can't, I don't have access to my inhaler, it's always in the back of my mind. Oh yeah, you are going to have to slow down a little bit. You can't forget about this because this is going to take some of your attention away from the task that you are doing. I try not to let it interrupt what I'm doing. But I'm always conscious of the settling in feeling. Like that chest tightening. It's always there. It's almost like it's a second little voice, like, "Pay attention to this, pay attention to this, this is still there, it's not going away." Depending on what I'm doing, where I'm at, I continue the task or moderate it and slow down a little bit to get back to the level of normal, I guess. It's definitely when I take—I call it "test breathing" almost like—okay, I haven't actually put a scale to it, but I guess I can put a mental scale to it and know when I'm at a point that I have hit the inhaler threshold. So taking a deep breath and realize, I have time, this is not a big deal, this is pretty minor. A couple minutes later, kind of checking back in with it. Like, it's progressing a little bit. If I don't have an inhaler, I should look for one or maybe start thinking about asking someone or finding a cup of coffee or a quiet space to relax in, and then five or ten minutes later, all right, it's gotten to the point that I can hear it and other people can hear it. The wheezing. And then it's like, okay, this is serious and I should take an inhaler or immediately find an inhaler. Or if I can't find it, I need to find a quiet place to just close my eyes and just breathe for like twenty minutes.

And even then—it's weird because that doesn't make it go away, it just can bump it down a few levels and it takes—even if I get it away from the wheezy sound and feel, after twenty minutes of relaxing, it can take an hour to get to what normal would feel like. And that entire time I am very aware of my lungs and my breath. So it's a whole process. It's kind of complicated. But if I was having a really bad asthma attack and I knew it, I would use it [the inhaler] even if I had time to do the breathing thing, because standing on that edge of panic is not fun. Even if it is controlled. Being there is like—I would much rather just take the inhaler and know that I'm going to be okay. So even if I'm just in my apartment and I have a random asthma attack and I have plenty of time to just relax and not have to use the inhaler, if I know that it's feeling bad, I will use it, because it's scary. Especially if I'm alone. So I would prefer to use it.

In this account, Greg gave a detailed description of his "whole process" of attuning to his asthma, which involves feeling his lungs and also his breath moving through his body. He watches the clock too, so to speak. He knows that when his asthma emerges, he cannot continue his current task apace if he does not have his inhaler. He needs to moderate. All of this takes his attention away from whatever he is doing, so that he can attune to his breathing. His chest tightness is like a second voice.

Greg also employs what he calls "test breathing" to judge whether he has "hit the inhaler threshold." Is his asthma progressing, or have his symptoms dropped away? He uses this test breathing every few minutes to determine what kind of action he should take. Despite his attunement practice, where he follows his asthma as it emerges and develops, or diminishes, he would still rather use a rescue inhaler than breathe through an asthma attack, because "standing on that edge of panic is not fun." But he certainly knows how to stand on that edge.

When his asthma progresses to a point where he needs an inhaler but does not have one, Greg draws on a number of tactics, from asking friends and strangers for an inhaler to finding a quiet place to try to relax and breathe to drinking coffee—an age-old tactic used by many asthma sufferers.[18] But this is a process, and it is complicated. And it takes time—twenty minutes to make the sound of the wheeze go away, but up to an hour to feel like he is breathing normally again. Using an inhaler is far simpler.

Greg mentioned "control" in two different senses. The first time, he used the word to describe his asthmatic state in response to his doctor's recommendation—his asthma is under control when he is healthy. In the second instance, he referred to his ability to control his symptoms in the moment of an asthma attack. Given Greg's familiarity with his disease and different modes of care for it, I wondered at first if he had picked up the language of control from his doctor, or in a clinical setting. Over the course of my research, however, I found that the word *control* was ubiquitous in the responses of my asthmatic interlocutors, leading me to believe that it may be one of the best words available to describe this mode of care in response to disordered breathing.

Indeed, asthma experts recognize that patients use the word *control* widely, but differently, to talk about their relationships to their disease and its symptoms. The 2018 GINA report acknowledges that patients and doctors often mean different things when they refer to control:

> Many studies describe discordance between the patient's and health provider's assessment of the patient's level of asthma control. This does not necessarily mean that patients "over-estimate" their level of control or "under-estimate" its severity, but that patients understand and use the word "control" differently from health professionals, e.g. based on how quickly their symptoms resolve when they take reliever medication. If the term "asthma control" is used with patients, the meaning should always be explained.[19]

Thus, while the report recognizes the distinction, it encourages doctors to explain the difference to their patients (and perhaps even to encourage a shift away from this lay language of "control"). For breathers who know their asthma through attunement to symptoms—which may be quite situational, or episodic—daily medication can seem unnecessary because symptoms can be managed as they arise in most cases. Breathers develop control tactics over years of living with asthma, and these tactics may allow some to manage their disease effectively on their own terms, as Kevin suggested (see chapter 1). In some cases, individuals learn their asthma so well through attunement that they may "grow around" their disease, as Tim Brookes puts it.[20] For others, symptoms may become normalized and the disease rendered invisible.

These different ways of knowing, or assessing, asthma control stem from temporal differences. For breathers, control is anchored in the context of emerging symptoms, as a mode of care that responds to embodied symptoms and situations. In the context of future risk, the events and effects have yet to come, have never been experienced. Future symptom events are easy to imagine and relate to, but decreased lung function and medication side effects are harder to know in an emplaced, attuned way. Future risk is divorced from the asthma attacks that breathers experience and the emplaced knowledge that develops over time. Moreover, these modes of knowing asthma steer care practices in the moment, day to day, and over years. The breather may rarely consider this last time frame, from year to year or across the life course, which is part of the point of incorporating future risk as an analytic and assessment tool.

As noted previously, the GINA report defines the level of asthma control as "the extent to which manifestations of asthma can be observed in the patient, or have been reduced or removed by treatment."[21] Over the past two decades, treatment has increasingly involved controller medications, which are designed to prevent symptoms altogether by reducing airway inflammation and hyperresponsiveness. Not all people diagnosed with asthma need controller medications. Those with mild asthma—who experience symptoms less than twice a month, use a rescue medication no more than twice a month, and have not experienced a decline in their quality of life—might achieve control over their asthma through as-needed use of a rescue inhaler, monitoring activities (such as measuring peak flow), and environmental control practices.[22] Yet, the report notes, "chronic airway inflammation is found even in patients with infrequent or recent-onset asthma symptoms, and there is a striking lack of studies for inhaled corticosteroids (ICS) in such populations." The authors cite several studies to support their recommendation that "regular daily controller treatment should be initiated as soon as possible after the diagnosis of asthma is made."[23] Patients who wait to start ICS, for example, may exhibit greater decline in long-term lung function and may later require higher doses of ICS if treatment is initially delayed.

Asthma treatment guidelines, in other words, emphasize the use of controller medications, which need to be taken daily to work as designed. Medication adherence is implicit in the definition and assessment of asthma control. But this logic and practice of asthma control, as communicated by medical organizations like GINA, ATS, and ERS, is at odds with the perspectives and experiences of many of the asthma sufferers I interviewed, and with the constraints under which they live.

Rob, a white, working-class man in his late twenties, was typical of those who resisted daily medication. Like Greg, Rob cared for his asthma primarily through his embodied sense of the disease and attunement to its symptoms. Rob's use of medication was structured not by a doctor's recommendations but by the way his body felt.

> ROB: I'm somewhat forgetful [about using the daily maintenance inhaler] and I guess that's kind of on purpose sometimes—if I'm getting really good I will see how long I can go without doing it. And I will be able to feel a difference that is not unpleasant. Then I'll start using my inhaler again before it becomes something that hurts me.

ALISON: Can you describe that difference? When you know you need to start taking the Dulera again?

ROB: It's sort of when it—before it reaches that point, it's almost the feeling of having drunk a lot of milk or something and a lot of times you can almost hear like a whistle. You kind of sense that you are not getting all of it. Possibly from years of having to sort of self-manage. In high school adolescent years and you are sleeping over at a friend's house who has a dog—I'm allergic to dogs in an asthmatic way. Not like in a cute sneezing, red eyes kind of way. Like, I will have an asthma attack kind of way. So there has definitely been many, many nights where I have forgotten to bring the inhaler and I'm sleeping on someone's couch that is covered in dog hair and I'm just taking a lot of shallow breaths and breathing really, really deep through my nose and trying to relax as best as possible. Because it is kind of tied to anxiety and stuff like that. You get nervous and you can really talk yourself into a very extreme asthma attack. And sort of coming from that and sort of being in those situations, these days it just doesn't seem like that big of a deal if I was feeling tense, I can kind of do some deep breathing and kind of talk myself out of it. When it's at that sort of level. When it goes past that, it's just difficult for me to breathe. You can kind of visualize your insides and sort of like—I'm probably breathing through a sixteenth-of-an-inch hole right now. Yeah, it's very difficult, pains in the ribs, pains in your chest that are not related to breathing. And that whistling becomes a constant just, wheezing. It's usually when I lie down in the evening, that's when it will really come out. That's usually the reminder—okay, Dulera, I need to do this tonight. Or if it's a little bit more, I have to do the albuterol. And there have definitely been times where I didn't have the inhaler around but I got tea, tea will help sometimes. I have a lot of apples, apple cider vinegar sometimes will open you up. I have experimented with lots of different things. Calcium and magnesium are supposed to help. I was doing that for a while and then stopped because I'm kind of lazy. Anyway, you are supposed to do it twice a day. I have been pretty good about it lately because I have a bunch of them and I just got insurance. So I have been doing this twice a day and I have been feeling good.

ALISON: Okay, but it sounds like you've always had access to these medications. You said you try to go as long as you can without. Why?

ROB: Because I don't want to be on medication for the rest of my life? I don't like it. I would much rather—I suspect that if I did two shots of apple cider vinegar every day and took magnesium and took calcium, that it might be the equivalent of doing the Dulera. But in most cases I would have to be kind of backed into a corner to do that. I guess I just don't feel the pressure to get off the Dulera. It just seems unsustainable to take medication every day for the rest of my life. And I smoke, so theoretically, if I didn't do that and—the vitamins, the apple cider vinegar, exercise, which I don't really do— there is room to be better.

Rob moderated his use of Dulera—a combination inhaler that includes both a steroid and a bronchodilator to control symptoms and inflamma- tion—because he did not want to be dependent on prescriptions drugs to breathe. For Rob, being on drugs for life felt like being locked into a rela- tionship of pharmaceutical dependence, which was unsustainable over the life course. The prospect worried him especially because his employment and access to health care had been inconsistent. Rather than rely on a controller medication that he might not be able to afford at some point, Rob was more interested in testing the limits of his asthma by seeing how long he could go without using the inhaler. He was also interested in using nonpharmaceutical strategies to improve his asthma. If he adjusted his lifestyle, Rob reasoned, he probably would not need the controller medi- cation. Like others I interviewed, Rob used his emplaced knowledge of his asthma—his sense of his breathing, the feelings of constriction and pain his chest, and his experience with triggers—to anchor his attuned care responses, which included deep breathing and talking himself out of symp- toms in addition to using the Dulera as needed.

The 2009 ATS/ERS statement observes that "asthma control is best con- sidered as a scale or continuum" and that what counts as acceptable, good, poor, or optimal control is highly subjective. The authors note that "descriptors of asthma control such as 'acceptable' beg the question of whose perspective is being considered, the patient's or the physician's, and whether the cost (financial and/or drug-related side effects) of achiev- ing the desired level of control has been considered."[24] They go on to point out that the patient's perspective has to be the primary factor in the assessment of whether asthma is controlled or not. Perspectives on control may vary from breather to breather and may also be at odds with doctors' perspectives, but ultimately the assessment of control needs to take the patient's lived experience into account. To this end, the ATS/ERS state- ment recommends that clinicians use a health-related quality of life ques- tionnaire to quantify patient perceptions and also establish a baseline for the patient that can be used in the routine process of control assessment. While such a questionnaire may be helpful in making patient perceptions visible to clinicians, thus facilitating better communication between patient and provider, the questionnaire alone cannot improve patient education, lower the costs of prescription medications, or address concerns about side effects—all of which contribute to how breathers enact care, with or without medication.

Playing with/out Breath

> No one had ever thought of it, they always just teased me for having this cough that—I was just always coughing. Just a subtle cough and everybody would make fun of me. Like my Dad would make fun of me because I would cough and not know I was coughing. It wasn't like a sick cough. Like this tickle that was always in my lungs, just always there. I wouldn't know I was coughing and I was like, I didn't just cough. They were like, yeah, you did. It was just so reoccurring that I didn't even notice it.

Karen was one of the college students I interviewed in 2010. A twenty-year-old white woman from rural Pennsylvania, she had been diagnosed more than five years previously, when she was in the ninth grade, after her older sister suggested that her cough might be something serious (her sister was studying to become a physician's assistant at the time). Like other asthma sufferers, Karen described being chronically sick with bronchitis and strep throat, particularly the year she was diagnosed. After her older sister made the suggestion, Karen's mother took her to the doctor, where she was indeed diagnosed with asthma and put on an ICS. By the time of our interview, however, Karen was no longer using her daily controller medication.

> I think I was on that for like two years, but I didn't use it that much because I didn't like the effect. I didn't like the way it made me feel. I didn't like the way it tasted and it made me—it helped my lungs. I could definitely tell that it was helping my lungs, but it just made me feel weird and I didn't like it and I was bad at taking it and so—it's not like asthma was a prominent thing, it was just exercise-induced asthma and—smoke and stuff. So it was only every now and then. It wasn't all the time. So I was like, I don't need to use this. Finally I just told my doctor, I don't want to take this anymore.

Karen decided to stop taking her controller medication for several reasons. First, she didn't like the side effects she felt from taking it. While some asthma sufferers worry about unknown future side effects that might have long-term impacts on their health—a view expressed by Tyler, as noted earlier in this chapter—Karen did not like the way her ICS made her feel in the present. These two contrasting concerns with medication side effects reflect the difference between a felt experience and an unknown concern. Karen stopped using her daily controller for a second reason as well: she felt that her asthma was episodic, occurring only in specific situations or in the presence of triggers. It was not "prominent" enough to warrant daily medication use. The persistent cough that had led her sister to suggest she visit her doctor had cleared up over the two years that Karen had been using Flovent, an ICS. Indeed, Karen felt that the medication had "helped her lungs."

Karen had originally gone to see her doctor because of a virus-related cough. This, however, turned out to be only one variant of her asthma. The following spring, after she had been on Flovent for several months, Karen suffered an asthma attack during a rugby game. It was a very different symptom event, in a very different context, and she was caught completely off guard. The attack on the field was different from her persistent cough: she experienced breathlessness, an inability to breathe, on the playing field. With this attack, she gained a second diagnosis, of EIA. It was also on the playing field, however, that Karen developed breath control techniques, which eventually contributed to her decision to abandon the ICS.

> I learned to breathe in my nose and out my mouth and I was really impressed with how well that has really calmed my asthma down. I can prevent attacks just by breathing properly while I run. And I think that is why I kind of got away from Flovent, because I didn't like it, I learned how to breathe right, so I could—I was learning how to know that an attack was coming and would start to breathe better and would kind of hold it off longer until I got time to rest during the game. . . . I try not to use my albuterol, I don't want to be dependent on it, I want to get my lungs used to—and get myself used to—having my body control itself and take care of myself in the event that I really do need albuterol. I don't want to get addicted to it or have me just be dependent. So when I really need it, it will definitely work. I try not to use it as much unless I absolutely have to. When I'm exercising or getting a cold, I'm on it. I always tell people—they will not believe how many asthma attacks I have prevented, or feel like I have prevented, just by breathing in my nose and out my mouth.

Over time, as she has learned to attune to her asthma and her breath, Karen has orchestrated a kind of control that is different from the control that daily medication achieves, a mode of care activated in response to symptoms in place—and not just any place, but the space of sports and exercise. For Karen, it is not just a matter of learning to sense how activities or environmental triggers affect her breathing. Rather, her breathing techniques engage with the moment and its qualities. This is another form of attunement: she has learned to "be affected . . . moved, put into motion" by the interaction between her body and the world.[25] Her breathing technique is a learned response built on the emplaced knowledge that comes with experience of attunement. The playing field became a kind of training ground, a place to experiment with breathing techniques as a mode of care, a place to tinker. During team practices and games, Karen had the opportunity to monitor, engage, and tame respiration.[26] Physical activity became a space in which she could try different breathing patterns, slow down and rest, and learn when it was okay to reengage in activity.[27]

Shaun described a similar practice in which he moderates his asthma by moderating his activity—backing off or even sitting out to rest while he catches his breath:

> If I'm doing something like a pickup game or something, I can sort of pace myself. So if I start losing my breath, I can back off or it would be like I need to go out for a second. But I definitely notice a difference between when I use my inhaler and when I don't. When I use it I can just breathe normally. I will still be breathing very heavily, especially if I'm playing soccer or something where it's a lot of running. So I will be breathing heavy and my chest is pounding, you are exercising, but I will still be able to be breathing deeply and I feel like I'm actually getting ahold of that breath.

Shaun described this as normal breathing during exercise, as many people would. All exercise works the breath, but for Shaun, normal breathing during exercise means breathing on albuterol. He almost always uses it before physical activity. When he does not use it before a game or practice, he finds that he cannot "catch" his breath; it never reaches his lungs to give him the energy he needs to move. Unlike Karen, however, Shaun could not always feel disordered breathing emerge in a way that allowed him to control an attack preemptively:

> Normally this happens in the middle of doing something. Normally I will just be like running, running, running, and then, crap, I can't breathe. If I really pay attention to it and I have sort of—if I'm just running like out on a run and I don't have my inhaler, if I'm going up a hill or something and I'm pushing hard, I can start to feel myself start to lose my breath. My breaths get shallower and I start getting that tight feeling in my chest. So then I will just walk and the act of walking

for a few hundred feet, I can sort of just calm myself down and then I can keep jogging again. But that is really where I actually notice it and can see my limits. Whereas usually if I'm playing sports, it's just like all of a sudden I can't breathe and I have to go sit down. It feels like forever. It's not a huge amount of time. It's not an hour. It could be five minutes or it could be fifteen. I never look at a watch; I'm on my hands and knees trying to catch my breath.

Context matters for Shaun's EIA. If he is out on a run, he can monitor his breathing more easily than he can when he is involved in a game with others. He knows when to start walking, to "just calm myself down," as he put it—a theme common across many interviews: I need to stay calm and try to relax. In contrast, during a game Shaun's focus is on the game rather than on his breathing. Because of this, his attacks on the field are sudden and he is not able to moderate his exercise like he can on a run. His habituated response is to sit down to try to "catch" his breath. But it takes time to regain the breath, and on the playing field, the amount of time it takes him to recover "feels like forever."

All asthma care is emplaced care, care that is determined by how the body is situated in place and time. A term of French origin, *emplacement* refers to how a material thing sits or is sited. In military contexts, emplacement concerns how weapons are positioned in landscapes. In geology, it involves the particular positions of organic matter, often embedded in rich ecologies. Cultural anthropologist Harri Englund has described emplacement as a way of being "situated in specific historical conditions."[28] Joshua Reno, another anthropologist who has drawn on Englund's early work, writes that emplacement is the "material, experiential, and discursive process through which places are creatively elaborated."[29] Central to this conceptualization is the boundary making that happens through control practices. Each time Shaun removes himself from the playing field to catch his breath, emplaced care is at work; it is a response in which the breather uses his surroundings to care. Sometimes this care takes the form of creating a boundary between place or trigger and breathing body; in other situations, it consists of crafting a sanctuary in which to breathe.

Place factors into Greg's emplaced care practices as well, in particular when he works out. In contrast to others, Greg expressed having a "good" association with exercise-induced asthma symptoms because they happen in a controlled context:

My association with exercise-induced asthma is almost good with the asthma attack. It's like, I am working out and this is good and here comes the asthma, here comes the inhaler and it's gone and I don't mind it because I can control it and it's almost a good thing. That's weird but it's almost a good thing. But the allergy asthma is miserable because it makes it way harder to do that controlled breathing.

During my interview with Greg, he described (in great detail) at least three occasions when he did not have his inhaler. But in a routine context, like the gym, Greg had an easier time remembering to bring his inhaler with him. Because EIA is associated with physical activity, which is frequently planned, asthma sufferers triggered by exercise may be more likely to have their inhalers with them and often have a routine of using their albuterol before working out. In Greg's opinion, the gym provided an environment where he could control his breathing. The playing field also provided Karen with something of a controlled environment in which to learn how asthma symptoms emerge and how to respond to them using breathing techniques.

Historically, inhaler use has been associated with stigma, particularly in the context of physical activity. Using an inhaler has often been understood to signal weakness or ineptitude, or, alternatively, performance enhancement. This stigma was much less present among the younger asthma sufferers I interviewed—those under the age of twenty-five—than for those over the age of forty who knew asthma from an earlier era with greater cultural stigma. The asthmatic athletes I interviewed see inhaler use on the field as a common practice. Kelly, a twenty-two-year-old white woman who had been a competitive swimmer, commented that more than half her teammates had asthma. Indeed, my own assumptions about inhaler stigma in the context of sports were clearly out of step with today's norms. Among the college students I interviewed, seven of the twenty-four were intercollegiate athletes, and seven more discussed playing in recreational leagues. The stigma around asthma has clearly been shifting, undoubtedly with the growing prevalence of the disease, but perhaps also with the shared experience provided in the space of sports.[30] Not only that—three of the persons I interviewed reported seeing a doctor for disordered breathing (and then receiving an EIA diagnosis) only after an athletic coach requested they see a doctor during high school. This is precisely what happened to Karen during her rugby game—the coach asked her to see a doctor before continuing with practice.

Karen discovered something else on the field, however, in the context of playing rugby with other women: how to talk another person through an asthma attack.

> I have had people back home on my rugby team, the one girl had never had an asthma attack, she was just wheezing and didn't know what to do. I saw her and her friends were freaking out, they didn't know what to do, they didn't know what was wrong. I walked up to her and I was

talking to her calmly. I was like, listen, you are having an asthma attack, you are going to be okay. You just need to calm down and breathe. Listen to me, breathe in your nose and out your mouth. I just talked her through it and told her to breathe out everything out of your lungs, breathe in your nose. I talked her through it and it went away. It's surprising how when someone has an asthma attack, if you just talk to them calmly and talk through it, it will go away.

This was a dynamic I encountered over and over again in interviews—how others had offered care to an asthma sufferer in the midst of an attack. The situation that Karen described mirrors other stories related to me involving different kinds of caregivers: parents, teachers, coaches, and, perhaps most often, school nurses. Many asthma sufferers continue to use in adulthood the strategies they learned growing up, including breathing techniques. Greg told me that when he is without his rescue inhaler and senses an oncoming attack, he implements a breathing technique that he learned from a nurse in elementary school:

I was told to purse your lips when you breathe in. I remember the nurse telling me that, to breathe in by pursing your lips. If you don't have access to an inhaler or anything then you can purse your lips real small and take deep breaths. I don't know why it works but I still do it. I guess I feel more in control of that too. It's like, okay, I can now control it. And I also remember my mother always being like, Greg, you are having an asthma attack, you need to stop talking and just focus on breathing. And I have really nice memories of that, of my mom like, "Stop talking, sweetheart, and just breathe." And that is just a nice thing. So not panicking was a big deal and it made a big difference.

The asthmatics I spoke with often described breathing techniques as an emergent response to symptoms. Many reported that they learned these techniques from parents, teachers, coaches, or school nurses, and their descriptions exhibited striking similarities. Most reported some version of inhaling through the nose and then exhaling slowly, in a tempered fashion, either back out through the nose or through the mouth. Some interviewees had been taught these breathing techniques while they were having asthma attacks; others had adapted relaxation exercises they already knew from other settings. Alexis, for example, a white woman who was a junior in college and originally from New England, implemented a technique she learned from her high school theater teacher:

I try to slow my breath down. I actually learned that in my theater class. In high school. We did a lot of relaxation training techniques to get into character, and so I would always try and apply those to when I was having an asthma attack because I know you are supposed to calm down and that is what those techniques are for. When I'm starting to have the asthma attack, it doesn't feel like I'm getting oxygen, so I will try and do the relaxation training techniques, one of which is imagining a candle, a lit candle. Trying to control your breathing so that you don't blow out the candle. And that is what I will usually try and do. Or I will try counting while I'm breathing just to slow it down because I know if I start trying to speed it up, I will hyperventilate and probably pass out.

For Alexis, Greg, and others I spoke with, disordered breathing is, at a minimum, anxiety producing; sometimes, it is terrifying. People with asthma often use breathing techniques to help regain control over their breath and over events as they are unfolding. These techniques also help them to relax, providing another inroad to control. In this regard, asthmatics have tapped into care practices long used in traditional healing.[31]

Some of the asthmatics I interviewed also described their breath and body as unruly. Rob, for example, who was "born with asthma," had allergic asthma and went through periods during which he used a controller medication daily. Even so, he developed a range of techniques that would help him to get by in any circumstance—in part because he found that his symptoms were triggered by a range of places and exposures.

Yeah, I actually used to have an English teacher in the sixth grade that taught us how to do deep breathing. Before tests and quizzes we would do in through the nose, out through the mouth, as deep as you can go and as slow as you can breathe out. And I immediately put that to practice when I was in sixth, seventh, eighth grade, when it was really bad and when I was going around a lot of people's houses. And it totally helps. It relaxes you. Because you are having these shallow breaths, it brings in air the way you need it and it's sort of like—the crazy thing about it is you can't rely on your natural breathing cycles when you are having an attack. You don't think about breathing. But when you get tight like that, you do. Having a bit of structure helps. When I'm having an attack I have to consciously breathe either way. And if I'm already thinking about it that much, why not take as deep a breath as possible and slowly exhale for as long as possible.

The structure of this learned breathing technique helped Rob cope in situations where he either did not have an inhaler or wanted to avoid using his inhaler and signaling to others that he was having a problem. In this sense, Rob's breathing technique allowed him to pass as healthy in situations where he did not want to draw attention to himself. Emplaced control in such situations is not just about taming disordered respiration to stave off an attack; it is also about controlling self-presentation in social situations. As Rob put it:

> I'm already bad at sports and things like that from being asthmatic and just overall sort of with this group of guys that are hanging out and I just don't want to be the person who is like, about to die. So yeah, I definitely used a lot of coping strategies. I'm not one to draw attention to myself, and because my mom is so attuned to it, trying to hide it from her so that she wouldn't flip out became a huge thing. She would go straight to the doctor, that was why it was important to hide it from her, because I did not want to go to the doctor. It's like, she wants the steroids and nebulizer. The hard stuff.

Rob was concerned with appearing healthy not only in front of his peers but also in front of a parent who would enforce pharmaceutical treatments that seemed excessive to him. In this sense, his breathing technique granted him a form of control entwined with embedded social norms, both within the family and among peers (it is significant that Rob considers himself bad at sports, so he does not associate EIA with athletics). These care tactics have a circular effect, such that, as Ronald J. Maynard has observed, the better a person controls his or her disease, "the more it is hidden and the stronger are the social imperatives to fit in."[32] It is not just that drugs work as a technology of normalization; some asthmatics have developed ad hoc responses to symptoms that allow them to pass as healthy anytime their bodies scream.[33]

Because asthma is dynamic and multiple, and care happens at many scales, control can be directed to any one of several layers of disease.[34] When Greg and other asthmatics talk about control, they are referring to a cultural-material category that is different from what clinicians, public health agencies, and biomedical researchers mean when they use the term. In the clinic, the term *control* applies to measures of the extent to which a person experiences asthma symptoms, or not, and how such symptoms affect a person's life. For Alexis, Greg, and Rob, control means taming an emerging attack using a breathing technique learned from a caregiver—a school nurse or teacher. For them, control is an attuned and emplaced response to an unfolding disease event.

Asthmatics engage in multiple layers of control—control of breathing, control of environment, and control of medication use. These modes of control are different from the forms of social control, or power, that have been richly described by social scientists, who often focus on how governments enact control over populations.[35] Means of enacting control as a mode of asthma care may be imbricated with methods of social control—through discourse, biomedical technologies, policy, and structural possibilities and constraints. There are continuities and similarities between the modes of control that breathers enact and those that state actors design; the different modes are not always in opposition. The actions of asthmatics represent a hybrid of care, in which responses and practices may aim for control that is anchored in attunement and also in line with civic responsibility.[36]

Care Fully Controlled

Cynthia's house was immaculate: throw pillows perfectly placed, picture frames and tabletops without a speck of dust, zero clutter, and floors so bright I practically needed sunglasses. Maybe the house itself was just incredibly sunny. One wall of the living room had three windows plus a glass door, and there were two more windows on another side of the room. All were closed, however, even though it was a warm afternoon in early September.[37] Warm and sunny conditions, Cynthia explained to me, can easily coincide with poor air quality:

> If it's a humid day or something like that, you can almost see the air. And I will say to my husband, we need to close up the house—we open up the doors in the morning, and if there is a little bit of fresh air on a warm day we will say, oh, you know—but usually by about 8:30, 8:45 we close the doors. As you can see, most of the time, the curtains stay closed. I do not open the windows downstairs because we live on this street, and this street and the boulevard are very busy streets. We have buses that are up and down. We have trucks, we have fire trucks, we have everything, delivery, everything on that street. And because this is a wider street than a lot of the ones coming in on either side of it, people use this street a lot. And it's not like living in the suburbs. You can smell the air in the city that you can't when you go someplace else. So I tend to keep the doors and windows closed.

Environmental control practices such as those Cynthia described make up the pillar of asthma care least discussed in today's medical research literature, which emphasizes diagnostic guidelines, control assessments, lung function standards, and pharmaceutical treatments. Environmental control practices are, however, discussed and reviewed in much greater detail in the public health literature. Also, as became clear to me during my fieldwork, environmental control is something that doctors discuss

with their patients.[38] Among my interviewees who saw allergists, environmental control practices were part of their treatment strategies.

While some of the breathers I spoke with felt that environmental control was a worthy undertaking because it helped reduce the need for medication or helped with symptom control, others felt that environmental
control practices infringed on their lives or were otherwise burdensome.
Melanie was a white, middle-class graduate student in her early thirties
whom I met through the RPI study. She was originally from rural New
England but had lived all over the Northeast for the past decade, working a variety of factory jobs. She had developed allergic asthma about four
years earlier and was still learning to live with disordered breathing.
Because she moved around—from state to state and home to home—each
year, if not several times a year, she had found it difficult to make sense of
when and under what conditions she had the greatest difficulty breathing:

> I have noticed more recently some sensitivity around my cats. I have
> two cats. And I know I'm allergic to cats. I got tested for allergies and
> cats came up and I thought, well that is kind of weird, because I didn't
> really notice it. But over the last year, if I'm holding my cat, my eyes get
> really watery now. I'm actually having some kind of a reaction. So
> sometimes I will—now, especially, they are starting to shed and so I am
> noticing that when I'm in the house I'm all—I'll have like a tight feeling
> in my chest, but yeah. I hope I'm not really—I want to keep them—but
> I think—that must be more allergy induced because that is obviously
> connected to the cats. It's not anything I was really worried about, but
> I did notice it and I thought, that's bad. Imagine if all I need to do is get
> rid of my cats, but I don't want to. Yeah, they are a real stress relief for
> me and that's a huge benefit. Especially in school and—yeah, I get
> migraines too, a couple times a month and the more stressed out I am,
> the more I will get. Those are pretty debilitating. So if I have the cats,
> I think that helps.

A number of the breathers I interviewed described asthma in relation to
other illness conditions that they experienced and cared for. In Melanie's
case, disordered breathing was just one symptom among many, including
allergies and migraines. Stress reduction was more important than environmental control—which would have meant giving up her cats—in the context of Melanie's life. Generalized care of the self made more sense in a
sea of overwhelming responsibilities—which is how Melanie characterized her current situation. This was the case for countless breathers I interviewed: they could not imagine giving up pets, even though their nonhuman companions were likely making it more difficult for them to achieve

asthma control, as clinically defined. In these cases, comfort and companionship outweighed control, understood as a form of avoidance or boundary making.

While some asthma sufferers develop their own environmental control strategies through attunement or long-term experience with the disease, others adopt strategies recommended by their health care providers. Over the course of asthma's history, breathers have cared for their disease by attempting to eliminate or avoid the triggers for their symptoms.[39] Public health workers and doctors often recommend that patients get rid of carpets and curtains, reduce the use of chemical cleaners and scented products, keep the home clean to limit pests and mold growth, and stay indoors on days with poor air quality. The last three of these recommendations are very common in the context of urban and low-income asthma care, as I discuss in greater detail in chapter 5. It is also not uncommon for health care providers to suggest that asthma sufferers give up pets. Most doctors and public health workers I have spoken with, however, admit that it is almost unheard-of for a family or an individual to give up a pet because of asthma.

One general practitioner told me that if a patient comes in with allergy symptoms, especially seasonal ones, she merely suggests over-the-counter allergy medicines, such as steroid nasal sprays and antihistamines. When I asked her why she would not refer such a patient to an allergist, she indicated that many people are unwilling to implement the recommendations of allergists, so a referral would be a waste of time:

> Allergy tests are most useful if you have chronic allergies and could get allergy shots. But I only recommend allergy tests to people who would make environmental changes in the home. Like if you'd be willing to give up your cat or get rid of carpets. Otherwise, it just makes sense to clean your house and make sure you're not sleeping next to an open window during pollen season. The other reason to get an allergy test is if you don't want to take medication, which is the case for some people. You can try to eliminate triggers from your life. But that can be a lot of work.

Mark articulated this issue a bit differently. From his perspective, some environmental control practices were simply out of reach:

> Some of them make sense to me in terms of—controlling your environment is the wrong word, but arranging your life in such a way that you—where your interface with the environment is more under your control than someone else's control in some general sense. I understand the value of that. As a practical matter, where I am right

now in my life, I just don't know that there is a lot that I can do about that. I'm not really somewhere where I can say, well this is where I choose to live. Or this is how I choose to structure my time. I don't have that luxury right now.

Mark was thinking about environmental control in a context including but not limited to his home. He changed residences frequently for school and work; he did not always have much say in where he lived geographically, or in the conditions of the apartments or neighborhoods he stayed in. A person's ability to implement environmental control strategies often depends on many factors that the individual cannot control, such as matters of employment and housing, which frequently intersect with age, class, and race. The more power and privilege an individual has, the greater that person's ability to enact environmental control. Among my interviewees, higher levels of power and privilege also seemed to make it easier to use controller medications. Breathers who had consistent employment and health insurance talked less about rationing medications or about finding alternatives to pharmaceutical treatments.

Despite being very tuned in to the atmosphere, and also adopting environmental control practices, Cynthia told me that medication was the real key to stopping her asthma:

> It wasn't really all that long until they got it balanced and until she got me so that there was something I could take in an emergency. Yeah, I was always looking out the window to see what the weather was going to be and saying, okay, what is the air quality, or thinking to myself, how strenuous is this going to be? Should we do this or—it's just one of those things. I don't want to have an attack. And Derrick, my husband, used to always say to me, he doesn't even say it anymore, but Derrick used to say to me, have you got your puffer with you? I wouldn't even consider traveling without it. But I don't worry about it. There is a difference now because I know I've got it. It's very rare that I would even need it. Because I have the controller inhaler, so I don't think anything of it anymore.

Cynthia's situation is markedly different from those of the other asthma sufferers I interviewed. She has good health insurance. She has lived in the same house for more than forty years. Her partner helps with asthma care. She is retired and middle-class. She can successfully implement many of the recommended pillars of asthma care, including taking a controller medication, visiting her doctor for routine assessment, and controlling environmental triggers through cleaning and avoidance. Cynthia also clearly uses attunement to understand her asthma and determine what the day will be like; for instance, she takes a deep breath to get a feel for her lungs and assesses the air quality by looking out her window at the landscape. On some level, however, these daily care practices seem like leftovers from a time when Cynthia had less control over her asthma. Since the controller medication keeps her asthma in check, attunement and emplaced care seem superficial rather than central to her disease management. Illness experiences like disordered breathing, however, have a way of imprinting on the individual in ways that may be difficult to shed. Asthma may become embedded in layers of the self, which makes attunement such a powerful mode of care.

The three modes of control described in this chapter—breath control, environmental control, and asthma control—engage with the timescape of breathing in different ways. Breath control is immediate and attuned; it is a rhythmic mode of care that makes time as the breather patiently sits with and listens to the breath; takes physical space to focus, engage in self-talk, and relax; and tinkers with the body in an unbreathable world at a given moment. Breath control may be learned from caregivers, but asthma sufferers also develop breathing techniques as a mode of tinkering that draws on their experiences of past asthma attacks.

Environmental control involves physically changing the relationship between the breathing body and its surroundings, often through boundary-making practices. Environmental control practices may be informed by asthmatic attunement, such as when a breather needs to leave a space to avoid a known trigger. This mode of control often incorporates clinical recommendations, such as when a doctor suggests that a patient avoid certain objects, modify housing, or change lifestyle. Environmental control practices typically take place over a longer time frame than breath control, which is a response in the present. And whereas breath control is a mode of care accessible to all, engaging in many environmental control practices requires resources and social power, since these tactics often involve the assertion of control over an external situation.

In contrast to breath control and environmental control, asthma control is clinically defined. Level of asthma control determines treatment goals and benchmarks for disease assessment. Asthma control involves the quantification of illness dimensions, such as symptom occurrence and medication use, as well as lung function measures. Of the three forms of control, this mode is most divorced from the present, lived experiences of asthma sufferers because it includes an abstract notion of future risk. One way asthma researchers are attempting to bridge this gap is through the use of health questionnaires that connect the subjective experiences of breathers to asthma control standards from one clinical assessment to the next, thus creating a record of control perceptions and metrics.

All three of these modes of control stem from breathers' emplacement in time, place, and socioeconomic conditions, leading to different responses to disordered breathing. While the narratives and descriptions I have presented so far have focused largely on individual experiences, in the following chapters I show in detail how asthma and its care may be shaped by communities of practice, shaped by and dependent on infrastructure, and deeply embedded in changing environmental timescapes.

CHAPTER THREE

Counting on Breath

Making Time with Respiratory Retraining

The Buteyko breathing educator (BBE) at the front of the room encouraged everyone to relax. "Take a deep breath. Sigh. Roll your neck. Relax. Breathe normally. Don't try to reduce your breathing. Pretend you've never heard of the Buteyko method." Two dozen breathers sat in rows facing the front of the room, eyes closed, anxiously waiting to hear more about the "natural asthma cure."[1] Coughing and nose blowing punctuated the space, a nineteenth-century farmhouse. It was a cold, rainy March morning in Upstate New York, not the best conditions for those with asthma and allergies. Yet workshop attendees had traveled from Maine, Georgia, and even Florida to learn a breathing technique that they hoped could help them manage their own asthma care. While most suffered from disordered breathing personally, two or three parents of children with severe, uncontrolled, asthma were in attendance as well. These parents were looking for care pathways that could be added to their children's current pharmaceutical regimens. One woman accompanied her asthmatic sister, and one man came to learn with his wife, who had severe allergic asthma. In all cases, it was clear from participants' stories that the disease was having negative impacts on their entire households, not just on the individuals with asthma. The dedicated support demonstrated by the participants quickly created a community feeling, which lasted through the weekend.

The workshop group spent the morning listening to the breathing educators talk about the Buteyko tradition, the theories behind it, and different kinds of breathing exercises. Then the attendees had the chance to try the technique for the first time. Although I do not have asthma, I participated fully, sitting on the edge of my chair, hands on my knees, eyes closed, observing my normal, everyday breathing cycle. One of the BBEs cued participants: "In ten seconds we'll do a three-second breath hold, and then another. Take your thumb and forefinger and pinch your nose to prevent any air from entering. Your mouth should be closed. If you need to come out of the breath hold early, that's fine. Exhaling . . . and hold." Sealing off my nostrils, I waited, uncomfortably, unaccustomed to suspending my breath after exhaling. I began to panic at second three. "Take an inhale." I pulled my thumb and forefinger apart and away from my nostrils; I was practically gasping for air, so much so that my closest neighbors could hear the force of air against my nostril walls. "If you're gasping for air at the end of the breath hold, you're holding for too long. You shouldn't need to inhale more deeply than the relaxed inhales you took just before the breath hold," the BBE said. I felt a strong urge to take another inhale, to balance the deprivation and compensate for those three breathless seconds. Before the Buteyko workshop, I never gave much thought to how I breathe—how many breaths I take in a minute, how deeply I inhale, or whether I exhale completely. Most people do not think about breathing at all, let alone breathing as a timescape. The tactile breathing exercises forced me to think about, and feel, the time and space of breath in the body. I was startled by my panicked response to the first cycle in the exercise.

Breath holds, the foundation of the Buteyko breathing technique, are used to retrain the practitioner's breath pattern. BBT rests on the theory that asthma either stems from hyperventilation (rapid, shallow breathing) or *is* chronic hyperventilation. Breath holds intervene in the mechanics of respiration by bringing practitioners' awareness to the rhythms of their breathing and gently engaging them with the cyclical movement. When first learning the technique, students are instructed to start with breath holds of three seconds before gradually working up to twenty seconds and beyond. According to the Buteyko tradition, if a person is unable to hold the breath for seven to ten seconds without gasping for air, this indicates that the individual's breathing is disordered, possibly because of such health problems as asthma, allergies, sleep disorders, or chronic fatigue. As the BBEs continued to lead us through the breath hold exercise, I wondered what percentage of the population would struggle with a test that measured how long they could go without air, considering how many health conditions affect breathing. Of course, you are not supposed to be thinking of things like population health during Buteyko breathing exercises. The point is to focus on your breath.

Most of the workshop attendees who had disordered breathing reported having severe asthma. Some had uncontrolled asthma and allergies and suffered from symptoms several times a week. Others expressed concern over the current and possible side effects from the multiple prescription drugs they took to control symptoms. Mostly, however, workshop attendees were frustrated (in various ways) that biomedical treatments had failed them. They were desperate for something that could control their uncontrolled disease. They had come to the workshop to learn BBT because their symptoms had been increasing while their quality of life was declining. Those who had lived with asthma for most of their lives reported that old tricks and medications no longer controlled their disease; their asthma had changed or gotten worse, and they were sick of being sick. Participants who had developed asthma more recently, as adults, felt their lives had been hijacked for reasons unknown. Their prescribed medications were not working—and they had a lot of prescriptions. Everyone in the room could list at least a half dozen medications they were taking or had tried. When one woman mentioned "the bag" she had received from her doctor, the room erupted in murmurs of recognition: she was referring to the plastic shopping bag containing asthma drug samples that a patient leaves the clinic with after being diagnosed with asthma. Receiving such a bag of drugs is an experience familiar to anyone treated for asthma in the past ten years.

The workshop participants were frustrated, and their lives were out of control. The stories they shared over the course of the weekend showed a side of asthma not usually seen in those who have access to health care and controller medications: asthma in its severe *and* uncontrolled form. The success of prescription asthma drugs over the past four decades cannot be overstated—not only financial success but also success in saving and improving lives. Nevertheless, for some people, asthma drugs have not brought enough relief from disordered breathing. This chapter engages the perspectives and practices of asthma sufferers who make time for breathing in response to what they see as pharmaceutical failure. In my interviews with asthma sufferers at other field sites, suspicion, fear, and anger came up when pharmaceutical treatments were discussed, but these emotions were often accompanied by acknowledgment (and relief) that something had worked to control their symptoms. In contrast, at the Buteyko field sites, I mostly heard frustration. Indeed, pharmaceutical failure was, in some form or fashion, the reason everyone I met at these sites had turned to BBT.

Researchers estimate that 10 percent of the asthma patient population suffers from variants of severe asthma that cannot be controlled with current pharmaceutical treatments.[2] These variants have received much attention from the scientific community in recent years because they are very difficult to treat and their stubborn persistence suggests an underlying disease mechanism that differs from other asthma phenotypes. At the March 2010 BBT workshop, asthma sufferers talked about having attacks several times a week, with either little or not enough relief from prescription drugs. In our interviews, some talked about medication side effects or the numbers of medications they needed to take. But it was not just that the prescribed treatments had failed them. Most of the people I spoke with had searched high and low for alternative treatments. Acupuncture had failed them, as had herbs and air purifiers and all the environmental control techniques they obsessively performed. They had completely organized and reorganized their lives around their disordered breathing, but no amount of behavioral and lifestyle modifications alleviated their symptoms. Desperation came through in their stories, and a weariness hung heavy in the room. Not being able to breathe is exhausting. Caring for a chronic disease like asthma wears you down quickly if symptoms occur daily or several times a week. It puts you on constant guard.

The Buteyko method promised workshop participants order in exchange for submitting to a rhythm. In this, the technique is not so different from other clinical interventions: rhythmic therapeutic interventions are a tried-and-true response to disorder.[3] Rhythm provides structure. Most pharmaceutical treatments work through rhythm; for drugs to work, they need to be consumed at the same time each day, or at evenly spaced intervals, to ensure that the amount of biochemical product within the body stays at a constant level. Medications ritualize care in timescapes. In the case of asthma, daily controller medications, used at regular intervals, provide this kind of rhythm. While pharmaceutical adherence is an obvious example of rhythmic intervention, environmental control practices, including domestic cleaning, represent another form. Dust, pollen, and dander are well-known asthma triggers that can build up on home surfaces. Routine cleaning is a core part of environmental control practices performed in the homes of asthma and allergy sufferers. The Buteyko tradition makes use of rhythmic intervention in a different way, primarily through breath retraining exercises but also through other behavioral and lifestyle interventions that could be understood as rhythmic care.

Rhythm categories in therapeutic regimens take many different forms — hours, seconds, days, seasons, and years are familiar timescales.[4] Many scholars have described how these rhythm categories tie into capitalist structures that shape modern life.[5] Within medical anthropology and medical sociology, other scholars have shown how rhythms associated with pharmaceutical adherence serve economic mandates that demand that workers show up to the workplace on time and well enough to labor.[6] The sense of time cultivated through the practice of breathing exercises, however, produces a very different kind of rhythm. Breathing itself is rhythmic, flowing cyclically from one point to the next. The inhale and exhale, which circulate air between the external environment and the human body, create a timescape that connects the biological, chemical, economic, social, and political conditions that make up the breather.[7] Pharmaceutical care practices barely engage with breathing rhythms, and then not intentionally or overtly. The Buteyko technique can be considered a rhythmic intervention in a style that Maria Puig de la Bellacasa has called, in another context, "making time for care time."[8]

Time is always made, in one way or another.[9] Care time for asthma is characterized by sitting, watching, hovering, and moving with and befriending the breath. Care time works in relation to other kinds of therapeutic rhythms, whether treatment adherence or attunement to environmental conditions. In this chapter, I delve into the ways in which Buteyko breathing educators make time through breathing practices, practices that include but are not limited to tracking breathing practice and progress using both digital and pen-and-paper techniques, engaging with medical guidelines for respiratory rates, recommending breathing techniques that shift respiratory cycles, and engaging in the care work of instructing students and watching them as they relearn to breathe. Using the framework of care time, I will show how BBEs work with myriad timescales that have largely been rendered invisible by a focus on pharmaceutical adherence and pulmonary performance, which are the dominant timescapes for addressing breath in biomedical asthma care.[10]

Narrative Rhythms

The story of how the Buteyko breathing technique came to make care time is a complicated one. Most introductions to BBT begin with the story of Dr. Konstantin Buteyko and his theory of disease, a theory rooted in another timescape, one that has had difficulty fitting in with today's biomedical paradigms. This origin story—told by senior BBEs who were trained by Buteyko or his direct students—differs somewhat from teller to teller, but the elements are similar. Although most information about BBT (and the stories of Buteyko himself) has been passed on orally, a few authoritative sources exist, one of which is a 1982 interview with Buteyko.[11] The story presented in the interview mirrors the origin narratives that can be found in books about the practice and on the professional websites of BBEs. The repetition of the story—and the tinkering with it, based on context—can be seen as one of the many modes of care that BBEs perform. The BBT origin story is important, in other words, not only because BBEs use it to teach the technique but also because Buteyko's theory of disease engages multiple timescales and timescapes of science and medicine. How we think about things, of course, shapes how we care for them.[12]

A Ukrainian-born medical scientist, Buteyko studied medicine in the Functional Diagnostics Research Laboratory at the First Moscow Institute of Medicine in the late 1940s. In the 1982 interview, Buteyko located his theory of breathing in two stories. In the first, he told the interviewer that he really got his start as a doctor as a third-year medical student, working "long hours in front of patient beds," where he observed the breathing patterns of dying patients. It was here that he first understood the connection between breathing and life. In the second story, Buteyko described an acute event with one of his patients in which he asked the patient to take a deep breath for a medical examination. The patient fainted after taking the breath. "This accident," Buteyko stated, "determined the future field of my research."[13] He went on to explain that it dawned on him, shortly after this experience with his fainting patient, that chronic overbreathing might be causing symptoms in his patients, especially those patients suffering from hypertension, asthma, and angina. His long hours observing respiratory rates at the bedside primed Buteyko to pay attention to breathing in all his patients, thus setting the stage for his career and the development of BBT. This is where the care time of BBT began, in the detailed but also perhaps boring daily labor of observing hospital patients.

Like many scientists before him, Buteyko turned to his own body to develop his hypotheses. Plagued by hypertension (high blood pressure), Buteyko observed how his symptoms (headaches and palpitations) were influenced by the depth and rate of his breathing. He carefully monitored not only his respiratory rate but also the degree and extent to which the trunk of his body—shoulders, chest, and stomach—worked with his respiratory cycles and, by extension, how his breathing patterns shifted as he moved through daily life. In Buteyko's theory, the body itself is a timescape, with different strata of movement, connection, and rhythm. He began experimenting with reducing his breathing and found that breathing less decreased his symptoms to the point that they eventually disappeared. He then tested his theory on patients and came to the same conclusion.

Buteyko did not describe these early experiments in detail, but they were likely time-intensive. The embodied, felt changes that derive from slowing the breath down and breathing less do not happen at the same timescale as the relief delivered by a rescue inhaler. It takes time to retrain the breath and observe the changes made by BBT.[14] Care work in this context is slow. Breathing is an everyday, mundane activity, so ordinary and taken for granted that it is largely rendered invisible unless something goes wrong.[15] Attending to the everyday rhythms of breath requires a kind of watching and hovering, characteristics of care that have received a lot of attention.[16] Such pointed, diligent attention to minute rhythms can thicken the present, serving as an anchor point in the attunement practices used by asthmatics.

Buteyko was quite committed to showing how breathing rhythms matter for health, but he also recognized that the mundane activity of breathing would have to be presented in a scientific way that would bring it the attention it lacked in medical settings. "I realized that unsubstantiated declarations would lead me nowhere and took to organizing an experimental research laboratory," he said in the 1982 interview. "I needed to get data. . . . I needed to find interrelations, formulate them, and only then come forward with grounds for my ideas." The interviewer's questions prompted Buteyko to explain the science of his research and his method. Reflecting fondly on his 1960s laboratory, he described his experiments and results in the language of a clinical researcher:

> I created a high-class lab: we had about 30–40 instruments that registered almost all primary functions of the human body and gave out about 100,000 informational units per hour. The data was handled on the computer, which I called "complexator," and the people gave it a name "the medical combine." Materials about it were publicized in press, for example, in the "Izobretatel I Razionalizator' journal. . . . That was a unique machine, still unsurpassed anywhere in the world.[17]

Although Buteyko situated himself squarely within his medical field in the interview, he also delved into theories from other scientific fields and healing traditions—ecology, evolution, and Tibetan medicine. He stated that he had searched far and wide for research on respiration, well beyond his own field. The different timescapes and timescales of the knowledge traditions of other fields, which he could not find in "Western medicine," were reflected in his theory: "Western medicine does not provide any foundation for the theory of life whatsoever. There's simply no such theory. What is there is the theory of life evolution which may be put in the basement of the life theory. That's why I have to work on the evolutionary aspect of the life theory."[18] In Buteyko's view, atmosphere and breathing were the foundation of life, yet neither was given the importance he believed it should have in modern medicine.

Later, the interviewer asked Buteyko how his research had been received by the scientific and medical community. In responding, Buteyko pointed to a few contemporaries who had begun using his work and had built similar disease paradigms, but he also noted the hostility of his Soviet peers and rejection by the medical establishment. He described how his laboratory was dismantled and his findings mishandled and discredited by the minister of health: "That falsification was a good excuse to close

the laboratory. It was done on August 14, 1968. The staff was fired without any job offers, and equipment was taken to pieces." (A note inserted
at this point in the published interview states that the falsified results were
later validated in 1980 by the USSR Cabinet of Ministers Committee for
Science and Technology.)[19] Despite Butekyo's success in treating patients,
his theory and method were not well received at the time, nor have they
been widely accepted in today's medical arenas (an assessment I offer
based on the scant peer-reviewed literature on BBT in comparison with
other forms of asthma care).[20]

Perhaps in response to this professional rejection, Buteyko described
the science behind his theory and method at length in the 1982 interview. All subsequent publications on BBT have relied on this description.
Approaching the body as a complex machine in need of tuning, Buteyko
argued that many of the most common and pervasive chronic disease
conditions—hypertension, asthma, allergies, anxiety—are linked to, if not
caused by, hyperventilation. Breathing too fast and too much skews the
ratio of oxygen to carbon dioxide, such that the body gets too much of the
former and too little of the latter.[21] According to Buteyko, this can cause
all sorts of disease conditions, depending on a person's predisposition.
He described in detail how different physiological systems, including the
metabolic, cardiac, pulmonary, and nervous systems, may be affected by
an imbalance of oxygen and carbon dioxide. In other words, he argued
that a rapid respiratory rate and deep breathing are not only symptoms of
many chronic diseases but in fact also cause them.

Buteyko emphasized that in developing his theory he drew on very
basic medical science to highlight mechanisms that had become obscure in
mainstream medical paradigms:

> To heal the patient, you have to bring them back to the norm. More
> than that, my method is fully and absolutely well-substantiated since I
> do not propose anything new or unknown. I suggest we should measure
> [the] breathing of people with the named ailments to prove they have
> deep breathing, hyperventilation, and CO_2 deficiency (that's what we
> and our ideological counterparts have done in the works). That is why
> I suggest we reduce breathing, particularly its depth, to raise the CO_2
> level back to normal. I'd like to repeat it: to normal, that is to
> international standards that you can find in all clinics and functional
> diagnostics research laboratories. That's, basically, why my method is
> logical, scientifically proven, well-supported and harmless. The man
> can't die from reducing deep breathing to the norm. If we don't die
> from deep breathing, we can't die from putting it down to normal,
> which is clear to all.[22]

There is nothing new here, he declared; his method is merely a "rediscovery" of existing knowledge and a call to measure the ordinary—breathing. Hearing this description of Buteyko's theory, with its invocation of hyperventilation and the impact of the ratio of oxygen to carbon dioxide on cellular function, one might think that it would be simple to reconcile contemporary biomedical asthma management protocols, including pulmonary performance tests using peak flow meters or spirometers, with BBT. But pulmonary performance tests measure the force, speed, and volume of individual breaths. They are designed to measure peak capacity rather than ordinary, everyday breathing patterns. Pulmonary performance tests do not measure respiratory rhythms over the duration, the time frame, in which BBT works. The performance tests assess airway inflammation and obstructions that might impair lung function, but they are not concerned with the more mundane ongoing act of how a person breathes.

Buteyko emphasized that his method is harmless, and that the point is to return patients to "normal" breathing, as defined by international standards of respiration, ventilation, and pulmonary performance. In his descriptions of his breathing technique, Buteyko situated himself as a scientist of what he called "Western medicine." He nevertheless also offered significant critiques of the biomedical establishment. In the 1982 interview, he invoked insights from Tibetan medicine to criticize the dominant biomedical models of asthma:

> Before getting to the core of the method, I'd like to mention I think of two trends in medicine: the so-called "official" western medicine, and the oriental, particularly Tibetan medicine, the Jud Shi. The truth turned out to be on the Tibetan side: they have always reckoned all illnesses were caused by respiratory disorders. . . .
> . . . [Western models] neglect the main principle on which, by the way, the Jud Shi medicine is based, "The doctor may not treat until he knows the reason. Only when you know it you can guarantee treatment." Western doctors have now either stopped looking for the sources of asthma, angina, and high blood pressure or have faulty idea about them. That is why these illnesses are still incurable.[23]

It is unclear at what point in his career Buteyko began to be influenced by Tibetan medicine. What is clear is that he was interested in a holistic medicine firmly anchored in a theory of life, inspired by scientific and medical fields outside his own. In the 1982 interview and in a 1988 documentary film about his work, Buteyko conveyed his thoughts on ecosystem and atmosphere, human culture, and lifestyle trends. He was interested in what he called a "theory of life evolution" that could explain relationships between human health and disease and various earth systems. When asked what causes hyperventilation, which he believed to be the underlying cause of the chronic diseases his method is designed to treat, Buteyko pointed to modern culture—social institutions, diet, and sleep, but also pollution and war. In discussing these components of disease, he mentioned issues ranging from the scale of nuclear war and the way women are coached during childbirth to contemporary recommendations for sleep and the intensity of industrial agriculture.

Buteyko's narrative of the basis of his technique reveals two key ways that BBT brings together multiple timescales that are typically marginalized by today's dominant biomedical paradigms and practices. First, BBT theory focuses on how breathing rhythms—the rate and depth of breath—affect health. Contemporary clinical care does too, of course, and includes the measurement of respiratory rate as part of the assessment of vital signs, but patients and health care professionals alike may overlook minute changes in respiratory patterns, such as the difference between eight breaths a minute and eighteen.[24] The Buteyko tradition, in contrast, focuses on breathing exercises that attune to and befriend ordinary respiratory rhythms. Any person can observe, monitor, and experiment with his or her own breath, although it certainly takes practice to become comfortable doing so. The way in which BBT makes body and breath accessible to practitioners as well as to patients is perhaps its most important contribution.

The second way BBT brings together timescales is by allowing for conversations among multiple thought styles. Buteyko drew on research and theoretical frameworks from a number of fields and healing traditions. He put them in conversation and created a mash-up that reflected his own theory of disease and method of care. He showed that it is possible to draw together multiple explanatory paradigms for asthma. In doing so, he developed a theory that encompasses numerous timescapes and scales, from metabolism, respiratory cycles, and gas exchange to socialization patterns, environmental conditions, and the global atmosphere. Although the very basic, motley, and holistic approach that Buteyko used has not been taken up by today's leading asthma publications, which are dominated by biomedical research models, at the margins of medicine an international school of BBT thought and practice has been fueled by the global increase in breathing disorders and the limits of pharmaceuticals for treating them.

Relax and Breathe

My eyes are closed, and I sit with spine straight, but this time my hands rest comfortably in my lap. I am relaxed—a very different state from the one I was in two years earlier at the "Natural Asthma Cure Workshop." This is the last of my three sessions with Karen, a BBE. Each session has focused on a different technique that Karen uses with students. Her voice is soft and gentle as she guides me through the breathing exercise, not only cuing inhales and exhales but also instructing me to relax between breath holds by using visualization techniques. Buteyko himself emphasized the importance of relaxation for healthy breathing: "The nucleus of the method is reduction of breathing depth. How? Best of all, via relaxation of respiratory muscles."[25] Now a practiced student of BBT, I am able to sustain breath holds beyond twenty seconds by the end of a session. According to BBT standards, I am in the healthy zone.

Karen is pleased when we complete the set. I have made a lot of progress with my breath holds, yes, but I am also dazed and euphoric from our twenty-five-minute session. I laugh when she points out how I rushed into her office, frantic and stressed and ten minutes late. That frenzied feeling is long gone now. In BBT, stress is taken to be a principal lever of

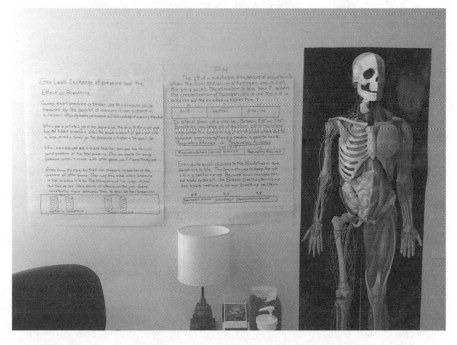

The teaching tools of a Buteyko breathing educator. I took this photograph in a California-based educator's clinical office in 2013. Instruction in anatomy and physiology, combined with embodied exercises, is foundational to this educator's approach to breath retraining.

hyperventilation and disordered breathing; relaxation is crucial for reset-
ting respiration. The move to relax in the face of disordered breathing
seems intuitive, so much so that many of the asthma sufferers I interviewed who were not involved in BBT workshops mentioned it as well.

As with the modes of care based on attunement and control discussed
in chapters 1 and 2, the foundation of BBT is embodied experience. The
power of the practice lies in the practitioner's embodied sense of change—
from the beginning to the end of a practice session, over the course of a
week, and over several months of using BBT daily. The changes can be
observed at the scale of the body, in its own timescapes, but they do not
happen overnight. Developing the ability to attune to and embody changes
also takes time. Andrea, a white woman in her fifties who had been practicing BBT for more than fifteen years at the time of our interview, explained:

> How do you develop awareness? Well, you don't just turn it on. You
> have to practice and it's like, at first you are never paying attention.
> And then it's like, 5 percent of the time you are. And so awareness of
> breathing, awareness of posture, awareness of how you are speaking,
> awareness of what triggers breathlessness, all of that takes time.

Andrea had lived with asthma for most of her life but had always seen it
as a "nuisance" until a life-threatening attack in her thirties put her in the
hospital. "There were a combination of elements that [were] making my
asthma worse. But because I had it my whole life it was just—I regarded
it more with impatience rather than concern. It was like, come on, I don't
have time for this." From that point on, however, asthma started getting
in her way, preventing her from doing everyday activities. Its increased
presence in her life, coupled with the "bag of medicine" she needed to take
to keep symptoms controlled, prompted Andrea to look for alternative
treatments. "I tried Chinese medicine, shiatsu, and acupuncture and herbs.
And I was seeing some change, but nothing significant."

A friend told her about BBT, which had recently been featured on a BBC
program. Andrea noted, "This was in the late nineties, and at that point the
web was not at all what it is today, the search engines were terrible." She
had learned about most of the alternative and supplemental therapies that
she had tried for her asthma through word of mouth and local networks.
After viewing the BBC program about BBT, Andrea went to England to
learn the technique from Alexander Stalmatski, who was a direct student
of Buteyko and had been authorized by the founder to train students outside Russia. After the training, Andrea told me, "I started getting better
and I was really, really impressed with the changes. You know, no more
symptoms, I didn't need the rescue inhaler or the controller medication,

and within a year I was off all the drugs. And that's when I went to New Zealand to become a Buteyko educator."

The embodied change that Andrea and other Buteyko practitioners describe derives from a personal practice that cultivates empowerment within the individual. Independence and self-reliance form as one befriends one's breath. As Andrea put it, "Really the biggest thing is the shift that people need to experience where they do take responsibility for their own health and [are] willing to put in the time for long-term benefits." The discourse of personal responsibility for health is prominent in the BBE community, but it is different in kind from the discourse of responsibility found in discussions of adherence to pharmaceutical regimens.[26] In biomedical contexts, the discourse of responsibility is about controlling disease, whereas in the Buteyko tradition, it concerns the individual's commitment to the technique for the purpose of personal healing. It is a subtle difference tied to distinct ethical positions.

Andrea told me that she tries to talk to each prospective student before the training begins, to explain the level of commitment it takes to see the impacts of BBT:

> When I suspect that someone is just checking me out and not really committed to doing the breathing exercise, I will actively discourage them from doing the course. Because we are both going to get frustrated. It's hard enough to stick with the exercises when you're committed. If you are just kind of like, well this is just my latest health entertainment, I'm not interested in that. I want to work with people who want to get better. And sometimes people need to have a real shift, mentally, before they are ready to do that. Because we have been so conditioned to pop a pill to feel better.

Daily practice is required—and not just once a day, but three times a day for twenty minutes or more each session. This kind of rigorous commitment is needed to achieve the radical and rapid shift in breathing patterns that Buteyko practitioners and educators alike talk about. But who has the time to spend an hour or more a day practicing breathing exercises? As many of the asthma sufferers quoted in earlier chapters indicated, part of the reason they take medication is that they feel they do not have the luxury of time to engage in alternatives, like breathing exercises. Mark, for example, could not structure his life in a way that would allow him to engage in alternative care practices. Rob, on the other hand, did not like the idea of taking medication every day, but he felt no pressure to get off his daily controller medications. He would have to be "backed into a corner" to make room for nonpharmaceutical practices.

Kim, a mother of three teenagers living in a midwestern suburb, developed allergic asthma in her forties. By the time I interviewed her, however, she had been symptom-free for more than a decade; she had been teaching BBT for just as long. She had gone looking for a treatment alternative because the medications she had been prescribed—an allergy medicine, a steroid, and a rescue inhaler—had created a host of side effects, which she attributed to the dosages. "I hated the medications," she told me. "I've always been a small person, a thin person. So any traditional drug will just really double do me, more than that." When she first learned BBT, however, the breathing exercises actually seemed to contribute to her stress:

> The asthma condition—it makes you anxious to begin with because
> your body's struggling to breathe and all that stress. And then to sit
> there and do those exercises where you're supposed to be really relaxed
> and quiet and still and breathing quietly and gentle. It felt like torture.
> And so I'm sitting there the whole time going, "Oh, gosh. Here I am.
> There's laundry that needs done. There are calls that need to be made.
> There's this and I just have to sit still and try to breathe." I was stress-
> ing myself out by trying to sit still and being able to breathe better.

There was no time for care time. In fact, making time for care added to Kim's stress—which, as described above, seemed to be competing with other forms of care work. But she stuck with the practice because the medications were worse, and the rhythms of practice eventually got easier. She did, however, have to rearrange her life to make it happen.

In the Buteyko tradition, the time commitment is precisely what is needed to retrain breathing rhythms. It is more than a matter of using an inhaler each morning and night, a practice that takes just a minute. Whereas pharmaceutical treatments are rhythmic interventions that get inserted into daily routines, breath retraining becomes part of the person in a different way. As Kim told me:

> It really does become part of your life. It's just something you just are
> doing all the time as life goes on. And that is what we want. It is tough
> to stick with the breathing exercises, that is the biggest challenge to
> Buteyko. So if people do start integrating it into their daily lives, that is
> the best way to see the best results.

Breath retraining requires making time and space for care at several scales—setting aside time for exercises, holding the breath and counting its rhythms, continuing the practice for weeks or months until respiratory patterns shift and asthma symptoms diminish. Making BBT work requires making time for care time.

Andrea talked about making time for care time in several different ways. First, she noted that students need to integrate the breathing exercises into their daily lives when they begin learning the practice. This is how the practice is designed to reset respiratory rhythms, through regular intervals of breathing exercises. This is also what she and many other BBEs describe as the "biggest challenge" to Buteyko—carving out the time to do the breathing exercises for a minimum of sixty minutes a day. But, Andrea explained, that is not something that practitioners will need to do as intensely for the rest of their lives:

> Because Buteyko is focused on your automatic habitual breathing, people shouldn't have to keep doing breathing exercises for the rest of their lives. Because you reestablished that healthy breathing pattern. Having said that, there [are] going to be periods in your life where there are bigger stressors than normal or you get really sick or you are moving or a new job or what have you, where you may have an ongoing stress for several months, which is going to impact your breathing. And so during those periods, what I tend to do is go back to practice.

By doing the daily breathing exercises and reprogramming their respiratory rhythms and habits, practitioners of the Buteyko method can restore normal, healthy breathing to their lives. But breathing, like life itself, is not a static thing. Successful practitioners reengage with exercises as the need arises, as life goes on. That, too, takes a kind of awareness that BBT is designed to cultivate, a different kind of making time to attune to the relationship between breathing and living. In fact, while the method is officially referred to as the Buteyko breathing technique, it encompasses many practices beyond breath holds, practices that cross various timescapes and scales.

Counting on Breath

In the first two chapters, I recounted how many of the asthma sufferers I interviewed attuned to their disordered breathing by sensing their bodies in environment and time. Beginning Buteyko practitioners adopt a slightly different approach to assessing their state of health, relying on self-performance measures rather than on their relationship to place and atmosphere.

The first step in the Buteyko method involves mastering the "control pause." The length of the control pause is a baseline measure taken at the start of the day, at the beginning and end of BBT practice sessions, and at the end of the day. As with other self-care technologies, such as the peak flow meter, the control pause is used to measure health and illness against both a standard set by the community of practitioners and the individual's baseline measurements. A control pause of more than twenty seconds indicates that the person has healthy breathing; a pause of less than twenty seconds signals that the individual is suffering from some kind of illness that is affecting the breath, creating a state of chronic overbreathing. Yet a control pause of more than twenty seconds does not necessarily indicate that the person is free of problems. Andrea, for example, described plateauing around thirty seconds after a year of intense practice during which she spent two and a half hours a day doing the breath hold exercise (this was during her training to be a BBE). Her trainer at the time suggested that something else might be going on in her body, something unseen that was blocking further improvement. Sure enough, Andrea had a bacterial infection, and once it cleared up she was able to register a control pause consistently in the range of forty to fifty seconds.

To measure a control pause, the practitioner holds the breath after exhaling until the first urge to inhale, typically signaled by spasms of the breathing muscles or contraction of the neck.[27] Buteyko described the control pause as "the time you can easily hold your breath for after exhaling. You shouldn't need to breathe more deeply after it than before."[28] As soon as the body signals a need for air, the practitioner inhales and records the length of time the breath was withheld. The control pause is not a measure of how long the person can hold the breath; such an activity would demand that the individual go beyond the point of air hunger, creating tension in the body and most likely ending the activity with a frantic inhale. The control pause should be measured in a relaxed fashion. It is a measure designed to be noncompetitive, nonstriving—at least that is what BBEs emphasize: if relaxation comes first, improvement will follow on its own. Improvement here may take the form of an extended control pause, closer to twenty seconds, or simply a reduction in asthma symptoms or other forms of disordered breathing. There are multiple readings of healing and improvement in the Buteyko tradition. The control pause provides a measure of improvement through the scale of time, but it does not demand speed, distance, or accumulation. The control pause asks, rather, how long can you sit there doing nothing?

Tracking exercises and improvement through seconds spent not breathing is crucial to BBT. As in most health assessments, numeric measures provide important information to students as well as to teachers. The progression of the breathing exercises can be tracked in different ways, digitally or on paper. At the March 2010 workshop, for example, the BBEs sold logbooks and timers for students to use in recording their practice. Other BBEs recommend mobile phone apps, which often include built-in timers. A typical log sheet is broken into five columns in which the student can record the durations of breath hold exercises and control pauses several times a day. The morning control pause, recorded in the first column, is the most accurate measure, since the body has been at rest and has not yet been affected by food, stress, exercise, triggers, or BBT itself. The next three columns are used for recording the morning, midday, and evening BBT sessions, each of which should be twenty to thirty minutes long. The control pause is measured at the beginning and end of each practice session; the end-of-practice control pause should be longer than the starting control pause.

Whereas the control pause measure is designed to catch the individual's baseline, the breath hold exercise is a temporally regimented practice designed to retrain the individual's breath pattern. The breath hold exercise begins with normal relaxed breathing for sixty seconds, followed by a breath suspension after exhaling. The breath should be suspended for a predetermined set of seconds. For example, if the control pause is seven seconds, the practitioner might start with breath holds of five seconds but work up to nine seconds by the end of the twenty-minute session. The inhale that follows the breath suspension should be a normal inhale, comfortable and relaxed. So, for example, when I started practicing BBT in 2010, I would breathe normally for sixty seconds, exhale completely, suspend my breath for three to five seconds, then inhale in a relaxed manner, and then breathe normally for sixty seconds again, restarting the cycle. This regimented cycle is repeated for at least twenty minutes, three times a day—first thing in the morning, sometime midday, and then again in the evening. The practitioner notes in the log how many breath cycles were done at different breath hold lengths. For example, my log page for April 17, 2010, shows that the morning session began with four five-second breath holds, followed by five seven-second breath holds, then five nine-second breath holds. Each breath hold was followed by at least sixty seconds of relaxed, normal breathing. The session described took me twenty minutes. I rarely went longer than this. Some educators, however, do so regularly, as a means to resist the culture of time scarcity that they feel is part of the problem of disordered breathing.

Obviously, BBT depends on the clock. Clock and body work together to shift breathing patterns. The clock is used to make care time at several scales. The clock tells the student when to practice, and the timer cues the student to inhale and exhale; it also tells the student how long he or she has been at the practice. Clocks and timers are essential for measuring the control pause as well as for holding to the regimented rhythm of the breath holds. The clock and the log sheet are tools that students use as motivation within their practice. This might seem antithetical to a practice designed to work against the compulsion to compete and progress, which can produce stress. In my conversations with Buteyko practitioners — students and educators alike — the mood was one of empowerment rather than competition. Seeing progress on the page and the clock is motivating, and the results are what keep them practicing. The danger here is that the temptation to privilege numerical progress can supersede the body's signals to inhale. It is crucial, BBEs emphasize, to inhale before the breath hold or control pause produces stress and discomfort. This is admittedly a fine line to walk when the structure of the practice puts embodied signals in conversation with time. BBT is a practice of care structured by a very specific relationship to time. Time directs the practice and the body.[29]

My instructor, Karen, does what few BBEs have been able to achieve: she teaches BBT at a hospital in a complementary and holistic therapy unit. BBT is just one of a range of treatments Karen offers as part of both inpatient and outpatient care. She also teaches BBT to health-oriented groups in the local community, free of charge. Like many BBEs, she is passionate about sharing the Buteyko tradition with as many people as possible. Her position at the hospital sets her apart from the majority of North American BBEs, who are predominantly small business owners. Most BBEs offer workshops and one-on-one sessions in which they examine disordered breathing patterns, share Buteyko theory, and instruct students in the practice of BBT. Ideally, Buteyko education happens individually or in small groups of ten or fewer students, so that educator and practitioner can focus on the unique patterns and minute details of individual habits of respiration.

At the last of our three sessions, Karen and I talked about the benefits of the practice. We discussed how the breath hold exercise cultivates awareness of physiology and timescapes using the breath, both during the exercise itself and over time with routine practice. It also cultivates a state of relaxation, which, as Buteyko emphasized, is crucial for breath normalization. Karen insisted that everyone needs relaxation techniques, whether or not they experience disordered breathing. And, of course, if done routinely — the daily rhythm is critical here — the breath hold exercise shifts the respiratory cycle and extends the individual's control pause. It is powerful for students to see how a daily practice like BBT can shift the rhythm of breathing. However, most of the BBEs I have spoken with have told me that few working adults have the ability to maintain the rigorous practice schedule demanded by the traditional approach. This reality is difficult for the BBEs, since nearly all of them attribute dramatic improvements in their lives to the breath hold practice. They became free of asthma symptoms and were able to reduce or stop taking medications, yes, but they also experienced other changes. Disordered breathing stopped running their lives. They were less prone to worry and fear, canceled fewer social engagements, and enjoyed more activities than they did before they began practicing BBT. Their sleep was better, too, and their quality of life improved overall. This personal experience with breathing, a new kind of relationship with its rhythms and place in the body, has led many BBEs to begin innovating with the tradition to make BBT more widely accessible. This has meant making a kind of care time that is different from the kind Buteyko used in his clinical practice.

Making Time for Care Time

More than fifty BBEs packed the conference room at a Boston hotel, seated at rows of tables facing the front of the room, where Patrick McKeown was giving a presentation. Most had conference materials scattered in front of them—annual reports, printouts of presentation slides, presenter bios, and articles that conveyed the most up-to-date standards of BBT practice. Many were taking notes. It was the first morning of the annual four-day meeting of the Buteyko Breathing Educators Association (BBEA). McKeown had been presenting the latest research in respiratory medicine and sports performance for nearly two hours, engaging the audience and his material with the kind of energy found in people passionate about their work. Indeed, McKeown, like many BBEs, had successfully treated his asthma with BBT more than a decade before. Now he was an international trainer and an author of several best-selling books. His demeanor was calm but sharp. He showed no signs of fatigue or slowing down as he presented case after case of research from a broad array of studies. Over the past decade, McKeown has amassed a huge digital archive of peer-reviewed research—an archive he was happy to share with me. His latest book, *The Oxygen Advantage* (2015), includes more than forty pages of footnotes, most of which reference peer-reviewed articles. He is a lay expert who has come to know the science well.[30]

For McKeown and many other BBEs, sharing information and helping to disseminate peer-reviewed research are critically important activities. Citing and discussing medical research that supports breath retraining is

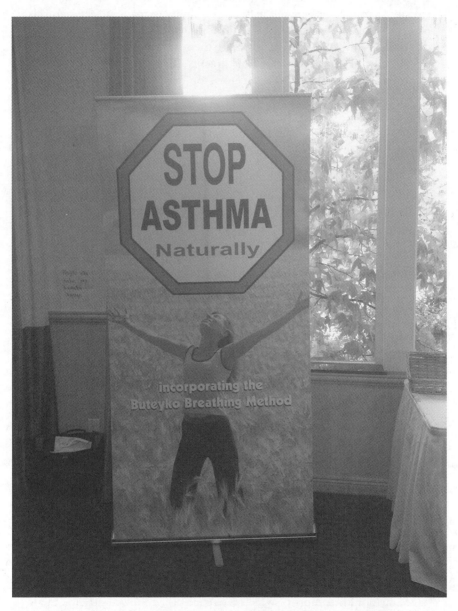

Display for Christine Byrne-Ralfs and Patrick McKeown's book *Stop Asthma Naturally* at the 2013 annual meeting of the Buteyko Breathing Educators Association, held in Seattle, Washington.

a core activity among the BBE community. Many BBEs keep archives of peer-reviewed studies at their disposal, often posting papers and reviews on their professional websites or making reference to them in marketing kits. Science citation is a legitimating activity intended to lend medical authority to traditions of complementary and alternative medicine in the broader health care industry.

The annual BBEA meeting stands as a premier event for BBEs, drawing participants and trainers from around the world. Each October, Buteyko community members gather to share the latest research, techniques, and organizational models. The annual meeting helps the BBEA, a nonprofit formally established in 2010, to execute its mission. Many of the founding members of the association received training in Australia or the United Kingdom and have long been members of the international Buteyko network, but prior to 2010, there was no professional organization in North America. Most North American practitioners were members of either Australia's Buteyko Institute of Breathing and Health or the Buteyko Breathing Association in the United Kingdom. Both of these organizations had been in existence since the early 1990s, when Alexander Stalmatski first began training students outside the former Soviet Union. BBT arrived and circulated in Australia, New Zealand, and the United Kingdom much earlier and more widely than it did in North America. The BBEA, however, wasted no time establishing itself as an active player in the international Buteyko community, holding annual conferences focused on training educators, sharing research, and fostering business development. The BBEA also sets global standards within the field of practice.

The BBEA anchors these efforts through its Training Institute of Buteyko Educators, with instructors certified through a separate organization, the Board of Buteyko Examiners. Both committees work to establish, evaluate, and maintain standards within the BBE community. This is particularly important in an international field, where lead trainers learned BBT through different people, at different times, and in different places. Six of the senior educators associated with the Training Institute of Buteyko Educators, for example, received training in four different environments: Tess Graham trained with Stalmatski, under Buteyko's direction, in the early 1990s; Patrick McKeown was accredited by Buteyko himself in 2001; Chris Bauman and Carol Baglia both trained with Jennifer and Russell Stark in the early 2000s; and in 2009, Thomas and Sasha Yakovic-Fredricksen learned the Buteyko method from Ludmilla Buteyko (Buteyko's wife) and Andrey Novozhilov in the Ukraine. McKeown, Graham, and the Starks are authors of texts that set standards of practice in the far reaches of the

Buteyko world (at least outside Russia). Despite BBEA's training standards, however, there is clear diversity within the field of BBEs. This diversity is visible not only in how the techniques developed by Buteyko and his students are used but also in how new techniques and approaches emerge from the educator community itself.

Different styles of BBT and breathing education, as well as varying beliefs about both, are juxtaposed at the annual BBEA meeting. One way differences are expressed is through debates over the traditional approach versus the modified approach. The traditional approach—that is, the rigid and uncompromising practices originally taught by Buteyko and his immediate students—encompasses the regimentation of daily breath hold exercises, mouth taping, and the lifestyle modifications that Buteyko recommended, such as a vegetarian diet, specific sleeping positions, and exercise regimens.[31] Proponents of the traditional approach, with its rigorous structure, assert that modifications to the practice reduce the technique's effectiveness. The downside, of course, is that most people find it difficult to fit this practice into their lives. As noted earlier, most people cannot carve out twenty to thirty minutes for breathing exercises three times a day in an environment where there will be no distractions. Yet the traditional approach requires that practitioners undertake exactly such regimentation to retrain and "normalize" their respiratory cycles.

Educators on the opposite side of the debate make the case for flexibility. Laura and Jessica, for example, two experienced BBEs with medical backgrounds, emphasize that BBT should be made accessible to those who are ill, and that making the tradition widely usable should be a priority for educators.[32] Both women work with chronically ill patients, many over the age of fifty; they care for individuals who have been hospitalized and diagnosed with comorbid conditions that may not allow them to practice the traditional Buteyko breathing techniques. In this context, both women have learned to modify BBT so that it meets people where they are with their health. While most BBEs believe that modifying the practice conflicts with the original teachings in a way that substantively alters the embodied experience—the exercises were designed to be a swift, rhythmic intervention for people who were very ill—the all-or-nothing stance has become unacceptable to many. For the advocates of flexibility, teaching people about the breath and giving them the experience of working with the breath in any way is more important than adhering to Butekyo's rhythm of care.

These two positions play out most visibly at the annual meeting during Q&A sessions. In their conversations with me, BBEs have implicitly described the traditional and modified approaches as occupying opposite

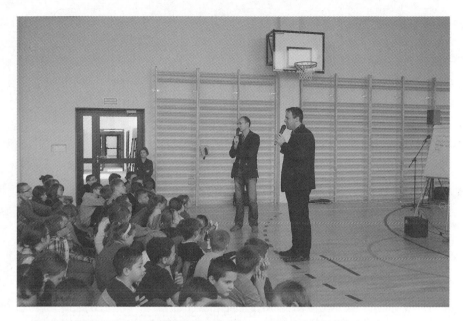

Patrick McKeown, a senior Buteyko breathing educator and trainer, teaches the Buteyko breathing technique to middle school students in Ireland in 2013. Photograph by Tsurk5vgr; courtesy of Wikimedia Commons.

ends of a single spectrum. What unfolds in practice, however, often seems to fall somewhere in the middle. One educator I spoke with—who had been practicing BBT for nearly two decades—typically begins breath retraining with simplified meditative exercises designed to acclimate students to the feeling of the breath and how to count it. This practice precedes instruction on the breath hold exercise. A direct plunge into breath holds, this person told me, can be terrifying for people who suffer from breathing disorders. Others, however, insist that the effectiveness of BBT—what makes it stand out from the sea of other breath retraining techniques—lies in the immediate shift in respiratory patterns achieved through the aggressive, disciplined pace provided by the traditional approach. For those in the traditional camp, BBT is first and foremost a rhythmic intervention that requires students to commit to a very specific timescale of care. The disciplined engagement with the breath is the key ingredient to BBT's effectiveness as a mode of care.

The appropriate timeline for teaching BBT is another issue about which advocates for the traditional and modified approaches disagree. As originally taught by Alexander Stalmatski and his students, people learned

BBT in a five-day, intensive program. Now advocates for the modified approach offer training workshops in weekend formats or spread out over the course of a month or more. On this matter, the experience of BBEs who have been teaching for more than a decade carries special weight. Like many senior BBEs, Kim travels widely to teach BBT, and she is a strong advocate for a modified, extended training approach:

> Not many people have the financial ability to just up and leave and pay all the travel and living expenses during that time. So we are constantly trying to figure out ways that we can make it more accessible, that we can train more people but not jeopardize the integrity of the information that we've got to get them to understand. . . . But how do we accomplish that when time is of the essence? People can't be away. And the hardest part—there's a lot that could be learned through webinars and online, but the part that's most important is working with individual clients. The hands-on clinical—this is this person's unique situation. How do I modify or apply Buteyko to get them the best results in the least amount of time and not cause reactions or different things that would set them back? We're trying to make it more feasible for people because we need a lot of people to learn this. It's just always been so challenging in the past because of all the obstacles and the time required and the costs required and it's just—we're working constantly to solve those obstacles.

In any given year, Kim guides about a hundred people through her ten-hour introductory course. She teaches the course over five weeks, with a two-hour session each week. It is designed to be the equivalent of a weekend workshop like the one I attended in March 2010. Kim explained that extending the introductory training across five weeks has a number of benefits:

> I work with people a total of ten hours. So they come for a two-hour class, usually five weeks in a row, and I give them an open invitation to come back to any workshop in the future if they need help. And, of course, they can telephone or e-mail or anything like that. I like to think if I do my job right that they're going to learn everything they need to know the first time and they'll get the results that they're supposed to. But some people do end up coming back. It's usually the elderly or people with multiple health problems, very complicated. And I know in Russia they're usually taught five days in a row. Very intense, like a crash course on Buteyko. Those are the ones that I find usually abandon it, because then there isn't anybody kind of watching over them. When I drag it out over five weeks, people get in a routine. They

get in a habit. They know somebody's looking at their numbers and following up. So they end up doing better and sticking with it when it's presented that way.

In Kim's mind, it is part of her role as an educator to develop relationships with students over time and to help them get into the rhythms, the habit, of BBT. Spacing out the training sessions helps Kim get to know the students, so she can "watch over" their practice and give them feedback on their numbers. As an educator, she keeps the lines of communication open—via e-mail and phone—and also allows students to return for a refresher at any point. I read Kim as extending herself toward others in a way that many caregivers do: "Again, I'm so committed to this. I'll do anything that I think's going to help promote it and get this message out there and get more people involved and help more people that are suffocating unnecessarily." The ethic of sharing the teachings as widely as possible, while also giving students the full power of the BBT experience, is a core goal of many educators.

When I attend the BBEA meetings and talk to BBEs about how they teach and support students, I see a form of care work happening—not only in the actions of individual BBEs but also at the level of the BBE community. It is a mode of collective tinkering with the care time made by Butekyo's theory of and approach to disease. Yes, there are experiments and debates, concerns and hesitations, but the overarching goal of the community is expressly to help people. This is an ethos that stems from the therapeutic (and ultimately healing) experience that all BBEs have had through BBT's approach to care time. The question, of course, is to what degree the rhythms of care time can be modified and still have the desired effect.

Breathing in the Time of the Inhaler

I learned of the Buteyko tradition from a November 2009 *New York Times* article headlined "A Breathing Technique Offers Help for People with Asthma." The article focused on a "natural" alternative to medical asthma care, a breathing technique that works both in the moment of an asthma attack and over the long term, as a sort of preventive shield. As described in the *Times*, BBT sounded like some combination of a rescue inhaler and a controller medication delivered through the breath. The article profiled a new breathing education center in Upstate New York where BBT was being taught to people with disordered breathing, their caregivers, and others looking to improve their health. The hook, however, was the article's description of the experience of a man with severe asthma, David Wiebe, who declared that BBT had transformed his life: in a matter of months, his severe asthma had become manageable and his overall health improved dramatically. These results were achieved naturally, without the use of drugs or dramatic procedures.

The author, Jane Brody, a self-proclaimed (and well-known) skeptic of complementary and alternative medicine, noted: "I don't often write about alternative remedies for serious medical conditions. Most have little more than anecdotal support, and few have been found effective in well-designed clinical trials." But this time, Brody made an exception:

> In describing an alternative treatment for asthma that does not yet have
> clinical ratings in this country (although it is taught in Russian medical
> schools and covered by insurance in Australia), I am going beyond my
> usually stringent criteria for three reasons: The treatment, a breathing
> technique discovered half a century ago, is harmless if practiced as
> directed with a well-trained therapist. It has the potential to improve
> the health and quality of life of many people with asthma, while saving
> health care dollars. I've seen it work miraculously well for a friend who
> had little choice but to stop using the steroid medications that were
> keeping him alive.[33]

She went on to tell the story of her friend, Wiebe, who was finally able to bring his severe asthma under control after suffering with it for forty-eight years. Wiebe had been forced off his steroid treatments after he developed degenerative vision as a side effect. The trade-off was severe: Wiebe needed steroids to keep his asthma controlled, but the medications that kept him alive were no longer an option if he wanted to retain his sight. Asthma sufferers who do not respond to standard asthma medications or who experience dramatic side effects, as Wiebe did, must make drastic choices that can have dire consequences for their quality of life. Some turn to off-label medication use, pharmaceutical cocktails, or experimental treatments.[34] Wiebe credited BBT with saving his life.

Modern asthma medications are easily taken for granted, and some of my informants—both Buteyko practitioners and others—criticized physicians' widespread prescribing of controller medications as an artifact of a global pharmaceutical campaign designed to put everyone on some drug or other for life.[35] At the same time, most expressed gratitude for rescue inhalers, which can relieve symptoms as they arise. Biographies of asthma sufferers from just a century ago, however, are excellent reminders of what life was like for asthmatics before today's medications. In earlier eras, those with severe asthma often led careful, even reclusive, lives.[36] Biographies of

French novelist Marcel Proust, for example, provide detailed reconstructions of how one severe asthmatic lived prior to the availability of bronchodilators and corticosteroids. Like many asthma sufferers who have come to be part of the Buteyko community, Proust searched extensively through medical texts and experimented with various treatments, but he was failed by remedies of the time. His asthma "dominated" his daily life, most of which he spent confined to his home. As historian of medicine Mark Jackson has observed:

> Proust constitutes the archetypal asthmatic, whose breathlessness and discomfort echo across space and time. Proust's intimate descriptions of his symptoms— "an asthmatic never knows if he will be able to breathe," he wrote to the novelist André Gide in 1919—bear striking similarities both to ancient Greek and medieval accounts of asthma many centuries earlier and to recent surveys suggesting that, at the turn of the millennium, many asthmatics continue to suffer from severe attacks that prevent them from speaking or make them fear for their lives.[37]

Rescue inhalers and controller medications have saved many lives and made the world more breathable for many more. But not all who suffer from disordered breathing have experienced such pharmaceutical success. So powerful and potent are the benefits of medications that the limitations and failures of asthma drugs—not to mention their costs and side effects, known and unknown—are rarely found in representations of asthma.[38] And yet some asthma sufferers experience precisely this failure: they either cannot take or cannot afford the available medications, or their condition does not respond to pharmaceuticals.[39]

The internet has made it possible for people with untreated diseases, including asthma, to learn how others manage their conditions. Wiebe discovered the Buteyko tradition online, as have many others. More than half the Buteyko educators interviewed for this project learned about Buteyko while conducting internet searches for alternative, natural, or holistic asthma treatments. Keith, a BBE who had been practicing the technique for just over ten years at the time of our interview, said that the internet made it possible for him to find alternatives: "I began researching and looking right around the advent of the internet. And then I began looking at treatments around the world for asthma, and that's how I stumbled upon Buteyko—online." Keith had lived with severe allergic asthma since he was a teenager. Most of the time, he struggled to control his symptoms, even with allergy shots, a controller medication, and a rescue inhaler. Living in a small town in the rural Midwest, Keith told me, he probably never would have found Buteyko without the internet. Now, in his mid-thirties, it had been years since he had experienced allergy or asthma symptoms. In more recent years, his practice has been supported in new ways through the online community that has emerged around BBEA, which includes e-mail lists, quarterly publications, and virtual classes.

BBT's availability in the United States grew as access to the internet expanded in the late 1990s. Nevertheless, twenty years later, it can still be difficult for American asthma sufferers to find BBEs. In early 2017, BBEA, which covers all of North America, had just over a hundred certified members. Many educators are clustered in specific regions—the West Coast and the Northeast dominate the U.S. BBE map, for example. Despite the growth of the BBE community, BBT still does not have the kind of mainstream visibility in North America that educators believe it should have. This is particularly evident given BBT's status in other countries, where it is taught in medical schools (Russia), covered by health insurance (Australia), used in hospitals (New Zealand), and recommended by professional medical associations (the United Kingdom).[40] Many U.S.-based BBEs hoped that Brody's 2009 article would generate exactly the kind of publicity the technique needed to go mainstream. In the United Kingdom and Australia, BBT took off after similar media coverage. Cultural visibility, I was told, can translate into demands on the medical establishment to engage with alternative treatments. And, by extension, such engagement can encourage clinical trials. "It just needs a spark like that . . . a really quality interview with some good testimonials on a national show. I think that would do wonders," Michelle, another midwestern BBE, told me.[41]

By all accounts, however, the *New York Times* article did not have the desired effect (although it did bring attention to the specific Buteyko center featured in the article). In fact, the BBEs I interviewed who have practiced in the United States for five years or more reported that business actually slowed a bit in 2013 and 2014, instead of increasing as had been predicted. The number of asthma sufferers seeking instruction has dropped; in some cases, people with asthma no longer account for the majority of people attending BBT workshops. Instead, a growing number of those registering for workshops, training, and one-on-one sessions suffer from sleep apnea and allergies.[42] BBEs also report that health and wellness workers who specialize in conditions other than asthma are increasingly interested in their work. Bodyworkers, dental professionals, and sleep therapists are among the fast-growing constituencies in the Buteyko community. The change in the BBT student base signals a broader shift in health culture. Breathing is increasingly recognized as a crucial pathway for working with the body, but mostly in health and wellness fields where breathing already has a presence as an object of concern and care.[43] Unfortunately, such recognition and interest do not seem to have taken hold in asthma care arenas.

There is little evidence of enthusiasm for breath retraining in mainstream asthma treatment arenas in the United States. Research trends that focus on molecular approaches keep physiological dynamics out of the mainstream view. The vast majority of asthma health professionals continue to focus on controlling asthma through adherence to prescription medications. The treatment paradigms that inform these approaches largely ignore the everyday rhythms of breathing. The focus in treatment research is on how past events, such as environmental exposures, and inherited traits produce specific disease variants, and on how pharmaceuticals can more efficiently control them in the future.

When I asked Gary, another BBE, why BBT has yet to take off in the United States, he replied, "Food and fitness are huge industries, but there are products attached to them." There is not much money to be made out of, or from, breathing. A recent review of the field of breath retraining research similarly highlights the absence of institutional resources: "Unlike pharmacology, there is no industry supporter."[44] The absence of social and scientific capital limits the growth of breath retraining in clinical research and, by extension, in health care institutions.[45] Perhaps a compromise can be made, one that keeps various modes of care in the mix. That is where educator Kim has set her sights: "That's really my goal, that anytime anyone is prescribed an inhaler, they should be sent for a breathing lesson."

CHAPTER FOUR

The Datafication of Care

Datafication is the translation of "qualitative aspects of life into quantified data."[1] The trend toward datafication has been lauded in various pockets of the health care field, and it is increasingly a driver of medical technology and health care policy innovation in the United States. Sometimes the effects of datafication are easy to see, but sometimes they are overlooked, no doubt because they are becoming ubiquitous and are also often hidden from view. Datafication happens across various scales and registers. In the context of asthma care, data are imagined to be a means through which patients, doctors, researchers, and even eventually policy makers can better address the disease. Data on illness events, medication use, and lung function, for example, can help breathers and their doctors work more effectively toward asthma control. And in the context of the asthma epidemic, care data made collective through public health research can lend insight into unbreathable built and natural environments. Data can care for asthma, in other words, not only by helping individuals control their disease through treatment adherence—which is often the starting point for the design of mobile apps for asthma care—but also through broader public health initiatives that collect the data of many individuals to situate populations in time and place. Asthma care apps can work at the scale of the individual as well as at the scale of populations in new ways. This is the claim of Propeller Health, one of the oldest and most successful asthma care application projects on record.

A brief video created by Propeller Health to explain the Propeller app begins with a view of Earth from space and a digital pinpoint moving across the screen. It zooms in and out of locations where people are using inhalers. It then cuts to a brief schematic shot of a GPS sensor before moving back to a map that connects inhaler, sensor, and the location of use. The voice-over walks viewers through the implications of the project:

Each day millions of Americans carry and use inhalers to relieve asthma and COPD symptoms. How often a person uses their inhaler indicates how well their disease is managed. The Propeller sensor is a small device that attaches easily to most inhalers. It automatically determines the time and location when the inhaler is used, *because revealing where people use their inhalers provides valuable clues about environmental exposures that cause attacks.* Our FDA-cleared mobile solution helps patients, physicians, and public health agencies systematically manage COPD and asthma in real time. So they can put the latest information to work to better understand and control respiratory disease.[2]

Zooming out again, the video shows a satellite collecting data signals from all the Propeller sensors, which are marking real-time use of rescue inhalers across the United States. Cutting to a map of San Francisco's Mission District, the video shows the locations of all inhalers being used in the sample neighborhood. Superimposed over the locations are areas of orange, red, and yellow, representing local air pollution and potential exposure sites that could trigger asthma symptoms.

Next, two men—apparently patient and doctor, as one wears an examination gown and the other a lab coat—are seen in front of a desktop computer on which the screen displays the map next to a patient profile. The voice-over notes that the data gathered through Propeller sensors can be used in different ways: to help patients, physicians, and public health experts both systematically manage asthma in real time and "better understand and control respiratory disease." In forty-eight seconds, viewers get a sense of how asthma care can be coded in time and space, for their own health as well as for the greater public health. Care of the self could become a kind of collective care for the public good, thanks to emerging environmental sensing technologies and health informatics.[3]

Clark C. Freifeld and his colleagues have used the term "participatory epidemiology" in describing a half dozen public health platforms used to leverage crowdsourced disease data through GPS-enabled smartphones.[4] Although their article focuses primarily on infectious disease outbreaks, these authors note that Propeller Health (which they refer to by its original name, Asthmapolis) stands out as the only platform they examined that collects data on a chronic disease condition. Asthma is unique as a chronic disease because it can be triggered by environmental conditions shared by many people at once, such as in the case of the thunderstorm asthma epidemic described in the Introduction. Although Freifeld and his colleagues are careful to mention the limits of crowdsourced data for scientific research (because of problems like data verification), as well as the importance of maintaining existing disease surveillance systems, they laud the benefits of nonhierarchical, real-time, and environmentally situated information systems as innovations that could improve not only the health of users but also "the health of those around them." That is, such innovations are not just about the self but about the local community as well. Crowdsourced disease data "can augment existing public health practice, integrate with clinical tools, and help bring public health services and information to underserved populations," the authors assert in the promissory tone that has come to characterize the mobile health field.[5] Propeller Health exemplifies how a low-cost system can improve the "study of underserved populations living with asthma" by producing "a risk map for environmental triggers."[6] The idea behind platforms such as Propeller Health is that they can provide new environmental information that can be used to help high-risk communities. But can the data be translated into information that can shape public health policy in new ways?

In an early article about the project published on the University of Wisconsin's news site, project founder David Van Sickle underscored the scientific potential of using GPS-enabled sensors to track the use of rescue inhalers and gather data that could lend insight into the unknown causes of lung diseases like asthma: "Established risk factors for asthma do not explain its global prevalence patterns and time trends. Studies of epidemic asthma have demonstrated that understanding the locations where asthma exacerbations occur can help identify important new exposures."[7] At the time, Van Sickle was firmly situated within the discipline of public health, holding an appointment in the Department of Population Health Science at the University of Wisconsin–Madison. Previously, he had spent time studying asthma in India and on North American Indian reservations as part of his doctoral research in anthropology before working as a disease detective in the Epidemic Intelligence Services at the Centers for Disease Control and Prevention.[8] In founding Asthmapolis, later renamed Propeller Health, Van Sickle applied his deep knowledge about asthma in places where different kinds of problems with health infrastructure made treatment challenging. The platform was designed to help address such gaps, but it also partook of an emerging enthusiasm within the field of epidemiology for coupling the potential of GPS with personal technologies like smartphones. And, indeed, this particular project generated a lot of attention, not only in terms of press and professional praise but also in the form of awards and financial investments.

In 2015, six years after I first learned of what was then known as Asthmapolis, a search for mobile asthma apps returned more than three hundred results in Apple's App Store and Google Play. The GPS features and public health frames that promised to "revolutionize" asthma care in 2010 were less apparent five years later, having been crowded out by designs that emphasized treatment adherence and control.[9] Still, the field was multivocal: the burgeoning digital marketplace reflected various kinds of care logics in a wide range of designs. While some asthma care apps had a clear educational slant—for example, providing information about the disease to asthma sufferers—others paired features of illness journals with local environmental conditions to help users better understand their disease in context. Many of these apps featured data visualizations to help asthma sufferers understand their disease over time and in relation to pulmonary performance norms. Most of the apps featured connectivity, boasting of their ability to network patients and their care teams through shareable data. Collectively, these features were based in embedded assumptions about what makes for good care.[10] These apps subscribed to the idea that enabling asthma sufferers to see the trends in their data and share that information with care team members would help them to control their disease more consistently.

Asthma sufferers looking for a mobile phone app to help manage their disease will find plenty of options for both iPhone and Android devices. Although in my review and analysis I concentrated on asthma care apps for adults looking to track illness and care, users can also choose from educational apps, gaming apps, and apps that teach breathing techniques for asthma (like BBT). When I last conducted a systematic review of the market in early 2015, I focused on about two dozen apps that stood at the top of the field.[11] These platforms allowed users to track asthma symptoms, exposure to triggers, and medication use so that they could better understand the patterns of this often ephemeral disease. The top asthma care apps shared four characteristics: standardized tracking categories, options for data sharing, performance visualizations, and information about the local environment. Within these areas, however, they offered different options that reflected judgments about the importance of some elements of care over others. Some emphasized peak flow tracking, for instance, while others highlighted the utility of the asthma action plan or the importance of logging health and trigger exposures daily (or several times a day). Over time, I found that, despite superficial differences in design features, how these apps were embedded (or not) in existing chronic care infrastructures mattered for care, and for the data produced through the apps.

As discussed in the Introduction, medical anthropologist Henriette Langstrup coined the term *chronic care infrastructures* to describe networked health care systems: "Chronic care infrastructures are made up of various inconspicuous elements (medication, standards, control visits, doses, daily routines, sheets of article for registration and more) that tend to sink into the daily practices of patients and professionals." The maintenance of these infrastructures, Langstrup continues, "depends on constant work in order to remain durable—work that is going on 'backstage'" and is made possible by caregivers, for example, but also by various kinds of technologies.[12] Examining how asthma apps are intricately embedded in and also extend chronic care infrastructures forces us to consider the many different ways care data may be produced, understood, and used across health care systems—shaping how care is accessed and paid for, how asthma is studied and governed, and also how people experience and organize their lives.

In this chapter I explore the emergence of mobile phone apps for asthma care by analyzing product design and highlighting how different apps are embedded in health care systems. I present industry perspectives, using interviews I conducted with people who have worked on app development teams as well as press releases, news stories, and peer-reviewed articles. Specifically, I look at how developers, researchers, doctors, and caregivers talk about data in various ways as a means to improve asthma control. In my interviews and in media reports, I found nuanced differences among app stakeholders in how they talk about data and the effects of data for care. These different care logics were sometimes bundled in a single interview or within a single app design—a tension that is reflective of asthma itself. Asthma is a public health epidemic with symptoms that may be triggered by environmental exposures shared by members of local communities, but it is also a disease that is highly individualized and heterogeneous in etiology. Modern medicine often struggles to acknowledge and address individualized disease experiences, but smartphone apps are now being used to highlight the personalized contours of illness. These contours, of course, are often translated into clinical categories and leveraged to promote patient responsibility and adherence to medication regimens. But, while operating as a technology of the self designed to enforce personal responsibility for health, asthma care apps actually provide a rich example of how embedded we are in chronic care infrastructures eager to make sure asthma is controlled collectively.

The Value of Tracking for Care

When Steve's three-year-old son was diagnosed with asthma in 2008 following an emergency room visit for disordered breathing, the ER doctor prescribed a medication regimen and asked Steve and his wife to track their son's symptoms and medication use—routine advice for asthma care.

Steve, a software developer, soon realized that he could log patient care data more effectively and efficiently on his phone than he could using paper forms.

> At first I started doing that on paper and then I realized that, you know, the first time he had [an attack] we weren't at home. It would be great if I could do this on my phone. So the app came from that, really. Just a way to track symptoms and track triggers. In doing some research, I learned more about asthma because I hadn't really had any experience with it. I found that people do peak flow readings on a regular basis and stuff like that. So I just kind of tried to think of a way to make it convenient for us, really, but for other people to keep track of things too. Being able to have it with you and being able to have the data with you for the doctor, you know at checkups, and saying—oh, let me show you.

Steve's experience with his son's asthma prompted him to develop Asthma Edge, an app whose original and sole purpose was for illness tracking.[13] When Steve's son was first diagnosed, it was hard for Steve and his wife, Nicole, to understand the disease's patterns, when they might expect symptoms. Their son's doctors recommended that they track episodes to learn the disease, but Steve and Nicole soon realized that the smartphone framework had the potential to track numerous asthma dimensions—time and location of symptoms and medication use, as well as triggers—and also create data visualizations representing illness and care trends. More than tracking these dimensions, which would allow them to have constant access to records of their son's symptoms and exposures, the app would also provide a way for Steve and Nicole to share that information with each other and with health care professionals. In Steve's mind, having the data in shareable form was a critical component of care. This theme came up over and over again in my interviews with people who helped develop asthma care apps: tracking is not an end in itself but rather a practice that makes health care in the clinic more efficient for everyone.

When I interviewed Steve in late 2013, Asthma Edge had been available in the Google Play store for more than two and half years. In that time, Steve had learned a lot about asthma. Neither he nor his wife has asthma, so their knowledge of the disease was originally limited to what they learned from the local emergency department and their son's pediatrician. But to build the app, Steve had to expand his knowledge. He read up on the condition on the Centers for Disease Control's website and reviewed asthma action plans from his state's department of health. He also used information from a popular website on health and disease information maintained by the Mayo Clinic, a major research hospital in Rochester, Minnesota. When he announced the app's launch on Twitter, Steve asked for feedback from medical professionals and patients. Although he did not get much response through social media, feedback rolled in via e-mail and through comments on the Google Play site as people downloaded and used the app. This feedback became the primary driver of Asthma Edge development. Steve told me: "There were a lot of requests like, 'Hey, this has been great, is there any way we could add this to what is being tracked?' Or, I think originally I only had one symptom and one trigger and people asked if there was any way they could track more. We are [now] up to three."

Asthma Edge is a good example of an app created by an independent developer for personal use. Apps like this, designed primarily for personal tracking, were never intended to link up with electronic medical records or to collect population-wide data to support public health studies. Asthma Edge's original minimalist design reflected Steve's needs as a caregiver of a toddler with asthma who was very much learning the disease. He wanted to share this digital tool with others who were trying to understand and track disordered breathing. From Steve's perspective, openness and flexibility were important design features that offered advantages both for him as the developer and for other users:

> I purposely left treatments open-ended because there are always going to be new treatments, but I don't want to have to update every time something new comes out. And doses and things and stuff like that. So it's pretty much a free form and you put your own treatments in and then you can fix those every time you enter an attack or your treatment. There are a handful of base symptoms that [users] can easily customize, too.

Asthma Edge is a one-person operation that Steve runs outside his nine-to-five career, so a low-maintenance approach to development is important to him. But I was struck by the time frame in which Steve thought about his app: "There are always going to be new treatments." Speaking like a developer thinking about infrastructure, labor, and users, Steve assumed that his app would be around for some time. Long enough, that is, for new treatments to come out, and for his users' disease conditions to change.

While the design principle of openness made sense to Steve as a parent of a child with asthma and a developer, it introduced possible conflicts for other potential users, including clinical care staff and public health researchers. Health care providers and medical researchers depend on data infrastructures that prioritize comparable, consistent data categories. In contrast, Steve focused on providing an efficient, simple care tool for families. He had no interest in collecting data, connecting users, or advancing the understanding of asthma for public knowledge—all explicit aims of apps developed by clinics, universities, and tech companies. Nor, in his conversations with me, did Steve ever mention bolstering treatment adherence through design, a major objective of the vast majority of asthma care apps (as reflected in app features and their promotional materials). Steve's primary goal for Asthma Edge was to enable users to improve their understanding of their disease through tracking. This was what stood out most powerfully for Steve from user feedback:

> It's rewarding to get feedback from users that have used it, especially if it helps them visualize things that they may not have noticed about [their asthma]. There is a charting tool that will take your peak flow readings, for example, over time. It's got the green, yellow, red lines across and you can see how it changes over time. For me, since we don't use that with our son, just being able to look at a log from the past two or three years or whatever it is, and see, oh, last fall around this time he started having symptoms or something like that. I had a few people e-mail in and tell me, "I have had asthma for twenty-five years and this has helped me get it under control because I can see when things happen, or I can track my peak flow. Clearly problems from where I lived at the time or days of the week or—different things I was doing." I found that astonishing, that this little thing can help with that. Something like that I would have expected people to have a better grasp of it on their own, I guess. I don't know, if I had been living with it for twenty years, I would figure it out on my own.

Steve's comments reveal that he underestimated the variability of the disease. While a number of people who have asthma are able to figure out the rhythms and patterns of their disordered breathing, particularly in relation to time, place, and exposures, others are unable to reach asthmatic attunement. Tracking is intended to help all users achieve some level of predictability and understanding, no matter how confusing their asthma. Developers of asthma care apps promise that data will allow users to see their disease in a way that they cannot see on their own. An app's ability to deliver on this promise, of course, depends on algorithms, visualizations, and notification features that shape the user's experience. In my interviews with designers and even in exploring finished app design, I often felt that designers had underestimated the nuances and details of the disease. To what extent did app design need to reflect specific angles of the disease and priorities of care?

Still, some physicians extolled the benefits of straightforward tracking apps to improve patient care. Dr. Wilson, a physician whose clinic was based in a private hospital, had served on an app development team since 2009; he told me that tracking would lead to better care on multiple fronts, saying, "I wish they would take their medications like they take their phones around." A physician for nearly a decade, Wilson expressed frustration with his current clinical practice. He emphasized that technology would make asthma care better for both patients and providers. To my surprise, he did not see nonadherence as the most pressing problem in asthma treatment. Rather, he emphasized the lack of precision in asthma treatment. He believed the asthma care app he had helped to develop was enabling him to be more precise in diagnosing and treating his patients' symptoms:

> You have the physical exam diagnosis of asthma. You have a few medications on hand that you could use, but you really don't have a good way of sensing if the medication is doing a good job, if the asthma is well controlled, and if you can do something better for the patient. It's purely by history. And that ends up, unfortunately, notoriously inaccurate when it comes to people recalling how many times they woke up and all that, in the middle of the night. How many coughs. People just forget, they don't pay attention to these things, they don't track it. So what we did with the app allowed people, without even putting in any peak flow measurements, just to track it. The office visits are becoming a lot more productive. Because people either can e-mail it to themselves or bring their phone in. We don't need a lot of information. I can simply make that visit a lot more worthwhile by having this information on hand. Physicians really . . . pick[ing] a medication is guesswork. Because again, all these medications have the same approval process for the FDA, show the same 10 percent improvement. So as far as I'm concerned, they are all the same. But in real life they are not the same, some people respond better to one than the other. So by using this visual cue, one would know, by using medicine, are they getting better or are they getting worse? They would know it in real time. I don't have to wait weeks for them to get back to us. So this kind of streamlined the process, I had a lot more data to work with as a physician and it wasn't taking any extra time from me. Because I can't spend a lot of time on this, knowing how many asthmatics we have and especially with the future of health care and how busy primary care physicians are going to get. I need help. I need technology to help us digest the data and tell me, in a very quick, concise way, where things stand, so we can make the proper changes. Prior to this, it was kind of a guess—well, let's try this, let's see what

happens, kind of a deal. Now, I can put my finger on it and be like, you know, this didn't work. You are having more problems in the evening time, so let's adjust the time of the medicine that we give, the type of medicine. So I have a lot more information to help manage that patient.

For Wilson, the asthma care app removed the guesswork from treatment. It removed the necessity of relying on patient accounts from memory, and thereby allowed him to assess more accurately which medications seemed to help the patient the most. The app also reduced the amount of time he needed to spend evaluating a patient's progress—and time was important to both Wilson and his patients. When a patient shared data in real time, Wilson did not need to wait weeks for a report, and the patient was saved a trip to the doctor's office. Wilson could assess whether a given prescription had improved a patient's health within a couple of days.

In our conversation, Wilson emphasized that the way the data are displayed matters:

> The technology needs to make an interpretation of the data and analyze it. So raw data, we are wasting our time. I should never receive raw data, because what am I going to do with that? It's going to take so much of my time, wasting my time, to figure out what the raw data means. There is no room for that. The idea is using technology to analyze the data, and then let me know the analysis and then I can act on that. It will save everybody time. I see what they see and it's not rocket science, it's traffic lights. So it's simplified to the point that you can look at your data and know the reason—if you ever had asthma or have ever been diagnosed, you may want to know how you are doing. It's been simplified to the point that you can simply look at the graph and know based on—if you know traffic lights, you know how well you are doing. And so an app that requires a lot of instructions, they are getting it wrong. If it's an app, it should be intuitive. So it should be that simple. Basic, basic information. That is why you need a really good technology company to be able to do this, [so] that someone can simply pick it up and is into it.

Wilson wanted the app's output to be easy to use and intuitive for both patients and doctors. With everyone short on time, there was "no room" for interpretation in the clinical appointment. As Wilson saw it, good design, provided by a good tech company, would provide the answer to this problem. Good design was crucial for getting people to use the app, to get them "into it."

I wondered about exactly this same issue when I spoke with asthma care app developers. Would they be willing to use an asthma care app someone else had designed? App store analytics, including the number of downloads, make clear that there is a community of breathers interested in using emerging personal technologies to help them manage their disease. But downloading an app and using it are two different things. Not just any design will ensure the sort of ongoing engagement on which successful tracking apps depend. The details of design and function—the look, the sequence of questions, the choice of language—matter for technology use, and for care. These features are more often than not shaped by the specific health care systems and associated information infrastructures in which the apps are embedded.

Designing Applications for Care

We didn't want to just turn a bunch of papers digital. That was a mistake a lot of people made, was [to] just look at what is [on] paper and translate that exactly to a digital version. That is just a misunderstanding and misuse of technology. I mean, technology can do so much, why just translate that information? So we were very keen on using technology the best we could and not overstepping FDA's recommendation. We don't want to have the technology make the diagnosis, but just kind of push the envelope, getting closer to where the FDA would pretty much draw the line, what technology can provide for the patients, short of making the diagnosis and suggesting a treatment option, which is really the responsibility of a health care provider, not an app. So our idea was to allow the asthmatic to be able to take personal care and responsibility for their own disease by first of all visualizing what their condition is and they have done a lot of research on this and they have found that one of the benefits of technology is to see really—visualize how you are doing compared to everyone else. And once you know where you stand compared to where other people—where the norms would be—that actually added and increased people's adherence to their medications.

This perspective, conveyed by a marketing expert from one of the asthma care app development teams I interviewed, carries with it a number of aspirations for how personal technologies can be used for disease management.[14] First, the narrative suggests that the technologies can add something to care that pen-and-paper tools cannot achieve. But whatever this additional service is must stay within the boundaries established by the U.S. Food and Drug Administration. The app should perform care, but only up to a certain point. If the app starts doing the work of medical professionals, for example, it has crossed a line. This person drew that line at diagnosis and prescribing treatment. Instead of identifying new patient populations, this care app would enable asthma sufferers to see their disease in new ways by comparing their own disease status to that of other people. By enabling users to see themselves in relation to others, according to this marketing professional, the app would encourage adherence to care regimens and personal responsibility. This perspective contrasts with the more common tracking discourse, which suggests that self-tracking patients benefit from seeing their own personal data trends. According to this marketing professional, it is important for the self to be situated and anchored in relation to other data, other standards.

Asthma Check was one of the first apps I analyzed in 2013. Its use of asthma control assessment provides one example of how existing chronic care infrastructures are taken up in app design. In this app, design is shaped by the asthma control standards set by the Global Initiative for Asthma. Launched by a German developer who appeared to be contracted to develop care apps for a number of organizations, Asthma Check was free and well positioned in the Apple iTunes Store when I reviewed it. The "Check" function on the app's main menu walks users through a five-question asthma control assessment modeled on GINA's guidelines. The first question asks the user if, in the past week, asthma symptoms have occurred more than twice; the user answers by selecting "yes" or "no." The second question asks if the user has needed rescue medication more than twice in the last week; again, the user selects "yes" or "no." The same structure is used for the final three questions, which address limitations in daily activities, nighttime asthma symptoms, and whether "your peak flow readings coded yellow, i.e. less than 80 percent of your personal best?" The binary structure of the questions makes a definitive cut to reduce ambiguity: three "yes" responses are one too many, but two are okay. The five questions are each worth a point, but the user gets the point only by answering "no."

In Asthma Check, following GINA's control assessment criteria, a user's asthma is considered "fully under control" only when the answers to all five questions are no. The user does not receive a point for any question answered yes. The scores are color coded so that users can see at a glance their control history in their "Check" archives. Five points result in a green checkmark, indicating that the user's asthma is under control; scores of two through four produce a yellow checkmark, which means the user is at risk with poorly controlled asthma; a score of one or zero generates a red checkmark, indicating uncontrolled asthma. The results of the "Check" are displayed as a simple list, organized by date. But this information, once produced, stays within the app. The app does not perform any action when the results of the "Check" are within the red or yellow; the results are merely archived. Users can do whatever they like with this information. The responsibility to act on the numbers and related assessment is left up to the app user, the breather. The "Check" does little more than could be done with pen-and-paper tracking. The apps coming online today, by contrast, are much more likely to prompt particular actions when a user's scores deviate from the norm.

Some apps feature more detailed and layered assessment questions than those found in Asthma Check. Asthma Ally's "Evaluation," for example, asks whether the user visited an emergency room or was hospitalized in the last week.[15] It distinguishes between having symptoms and having a full-blown asthma attack. It also asks if the user forgot to take medication in the last week, and, if so, how many times. In addition, Asthma Ally includes questions about allergy symptoms and asks users about their environmental exposures. A daily "Exposure" log asks users specifically about a fairly limited number of asthma triggers: tobacco smoke, grass, air pollution, exercise, and contact with dogs and cats. It does not ask about exposures to mold, cold air, or viruses, despite these being fairly common asthma triggers, nor does it offer an "other" field for users to enter their own triggers. Asthma Ally also has a much shorter, two-question assessment that simply asks users to rate their breathing and allergies on a scale marked by facial expressions (as opposed to numbers). Users are encouraged to fill out the "How I Feel" log at least once a day, if not more often.

Other apps allow for more customization. Asthma Storylines, for instance, allows users to add specific symptoms and triggers to a list of standard options, striking a balance between customization and data consistency. Launched in early 2017, Asthma Storylines almost feels more like a lifestyle app than a health app. It features a series of about a dozen tiles where users can enter a broad range of health data, including information on daily mood, vitals, and medical appointments, as well as standard asthma tracking categories. It also offers two journaling spaces where users can reflect on doctor visits and self-care. A function called "Healthy Doses" generates inspirational quotations related to love, mindfulness, optimism, and gratitude. The app tells the user, "Collect a dose of healthy wisdom for your mind and spirit." Each of the app tiles generates a user "storyline" based on the entered data. The visualizations are presented primarily in graph or calendar form.

Asthma Storylines also creates a community feel through user groups, polls, and a link to the Self Care Movement website, where people share their stories and learn about others. This feature reflects the goals of the Allergy and Asthma Network, the U.S.-based nonprofit patient education

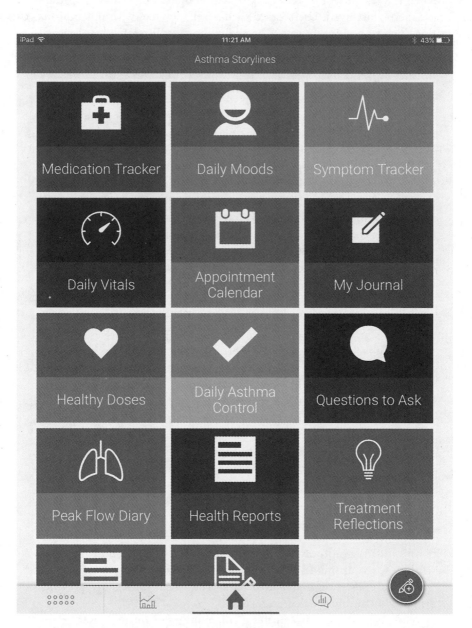

iPad screenshot of the main menu for Asthma Storylines.

and advocacy organization for asthma that developed the Asthma Story-lines app. The unique functions of the app mirror features of the Allergy and Asthma Network's website: personal stories, reviews of research, care tips, and the message that asthma can be controlled through monitoring and medication.

Other asthma care apps explicitly incorporate the user's asthma action plan. In AsthmaMD, for example, one of the first things the user is asked to do when setting up a profile is to fill in the details of his or her asthma action plan, as prescribed by a doctor.[16] (Indeed, the user is asked to mark an additional checkbox at the end to verify that the information entered comes from a medical provider. Almost all the apps I analyzed incorporated messaging about the need to use treatment information provided by a doctor.) AsthmaMD translates the action plan information provided into a "live" action plan that the user can initiate when he or she starts to experience symptoms or an attack. When one of the three versions of the live action plan (green, yellow, or red—the user decides as appropriate) is initiated, AsthmaMD walks the breather through a series of prescribed steps to address the event, depending on its severity. For example, when the yellow version of the action plan is selected, the user is instructed to use one dose of prescribed quick-relief medication and wait thirty minutes. Thirty minutes later, the user receives a notification to check back in. At that point, the user can enter a current peak flow reading or indicate whether he or she is still having symptoms. If so, the app generates further instructions based on the response and the prescribed action plan. If the red version of the action plan is selected, the user is instructed to use the prescribed quick-relief medicine and call 911.

AsthmaMD's live action plan is meant to address acute events. In contrast, most other care apps, including Asthma Check, are designed to perform daily or weekly assessments of a chronic condition and provide longitudinal data on daily care practices. Control assessments like the "Check" in Asthma Check and the "Evaluation" in Asthma Ally are designed to be completed once a week. Increasingly, apps prompt users to fill out weekly assessments, so that they can accumulate into a bigger picture of control, health, and care in the app timescape. This is how users are able to see their disease in new ways.

Most apps enable users to export their data to designated care team members, such as health care providers, spouses, parents, or even coaches.[17] In Asthma Storylines, for instance, users can create "Circles of Support" by entering the e-mail addresses of care team members, both personal contacts and medical providers. Whenever Asthma Storylines users enter data, they can select how visible they want the data to be. While Asthma Check charges users for a similar feature, most other apps encourage users to share their data and make this function as unrestricted as possible. Whereas first-generation asthma care apps—like Asthma Check and Asthma Edge—typically enabled data sharing via e-mail or download, newer apps allow users to add care team members to their accounts via cloud storage infrastructure. These apps operate under various kinds of data-sharing permission structures. Propeller and Asthma Health, for example, ask users to opt in to share their de-identified data with researchers who are conducting public health studies.

Compared with earlier asthma care apps, newer apps have a different relationship to chronic care infrastructures. When I revisited Asthma Check in the iTunes Store in mid-2017, the website link no longer worked. According to the update record in iTunes, the app had not been updated since 2013. Considering Asthma Check next to more recent apps, it seems visually outdated and lacks many features of the newer products. Asthma Check, like many of the earliest asthma care apps, was created by an independent developer to test the new mobile marketplace. These early asthma care apps often took the form of digital symptom diaries, some of which also layered in data visualizations and sharing functions. Asthma Check was not the only app that seemed dated: many of the stand-alone apps I initially analyzed in 2015 had not been updated in more than a year when I checked back in summer 2017. This was the case, for example, for Asthma Ally as well. In contrast, one of the only apps from my 2010 review to survive, AsthmaMD (in version 3.35 as of March 2017), was created by pediatrician Sam Pejham and a development team from the University of California, San Francisco. Pejham uses the app with his patients, and the UCSF team uses the data collected by the app to conduct public health research, so that AsthmaMD is effectively embedded in the infrastructures of clinical care and medical research. Propeller Health, too, which is partnered with many different kinds of organizations and agencies and has received substantial financial investment, had just updated its Propeller app to version 5.21.

The longevity of an asthma app, like that of most services, is related to its relationship to broader infrastructures, including both health care and digital infrastructures.[18] Apps designed and developed by organizations that use the apps in their own practices have a more stable existence than products developed by third-party companies that have little investment in asthma care or research. Arguably, developers who have some investment in the data produced by their apps—whether for the purpose of research or further development, medication adherence, personal technology use, or public health—back the most successful apps. When thinking about asthma apps as chronic care infrastructures, in other words, it matters for whom data have value.

Troubling Chronic Care Infrastructures

Cheryl, a twenty-two-year-old black woman, was born and raised in Philadelphia. She had lived in the same house for most of her life and grew up watching her family's neighborhood transform, an experience shared by residents of many Philadelphia neighborhoods, especially in the past decade. Our interview, which ran almost two hours, hit on themes that came up repeatedly in my conversations with allergic asthmatics. Our discussion of asthma care apps, however, stood out.

> ALI: What about an asthma action plan? Did you ever get one or use one?
>
> CHERYL: I actually have an app on my phone from Blue Cross, it's called Care Cam, where you check in every day with how your breathing is, and I don't really have an action plan. I have albuterol in my bag in case I need it.

I took a long pause. That was not a response I had been expecting. In seven years of formal interviews with more than seventy asthma sufferers, Cheryl was the first person I had met who was actually using an app for disease management. This was not for lack of curiosity—toward the end of all interviews I asked people whether they used digital disease management tools, such as health or care apps for smartphones. But up until my interview with Cheryl, not a single asthma sufferer I had spoken with said yes. Most did not see a need, reporting that digital tracking was unnecessary since they had a good sense of the parameters and rhythms of their disease from years of living with it. Others objected to sharing their personal data—especially their health data—with tech providers, citing privacy concerns.[19]

My interview with Cheryl—one of the last that I conducted for this book—took place in June 2016. In the six-year period since I had begun this project, the mobile health field had grown substantially, and not just in the number of products populating the marketplace. Health care organizations were also beginning to integrate digital platforms into patient care. Cheryl was introduced to the Care Cam app when she signed up for health insurance following passage of the Patient Protection and Affordable Care Act. But instead of asking Cheryl my planned follow-up question about asthma apps, I asked her to clarify whether she had received an asthma action plan. Hearing that someone had albuterol but not an asthma action plan was a red flag, of sorts, for me as someone who studies asthma care.

ALI: Nobody has given you one of these little one-page action plans?
CHERYL: I've seen it. I used to have one, I don't have one now.
ALI: Did you find it useful when you did have it?
CHERYL: I read it, I knew it was there. But for the most part, my asthma was under control, that's why I never took the action plan seriously.
ALI: When you say that your asthma is under control, what does that mean?
CHERYL: My lungs aren't constricted, I don't feel that tightness when I'm trying to breathe or I don't feel like I'm trying so hard to breathe and I'm just coughing. That's a scary feeling, when you feel like you can't breathe. It's scary. That's pretty much what I mean [long pause]. I have one, I guess, but I never use it. I should check in with the app on my phone.
ALI: Yeah, tell me about this app on your phone. How did you learn about it?
CHERYL: So when we did the affordable care insurance registration, since we have Blue Cross, they have an app that you can—I guess you put in your insurance ID numbers and so every day it asks you a couple questions, like, how is your breathing, and you can rate how well it is or how poor it is and so if it was on a scale of one to five, you gave it a three. Then they give you tips to check in with your doctor about it, make sure you are using your rescue inhaler. So it will give you reminders and stuff like that. It's also a way for me to monitor because you can check—there is a chart section where you can check how well it is or on days that you aren't doing so well and are having a hard time breathing. So it will also tell me that I need to have a peak flow number, I should know that number. I don't know that number. I don't know how to find that number.
ALI: So you use this app daily?
CHERYL: Mmhm. But I don't have a peak flow meter. I don't know what that looks like.
ALI: A peak flow meter?
CHERYL: Yeah.
ALI: You never got a peak flow meter?
CHERYL: No.
ALI: No one ever told you to use a peak flow meter?
CHERYL: They may have told me. [We both laugh.] I'm not sure. If you don't show me what it is, I don't know.

ALI: Did you ever get one, do you think?

CHERYL: I've seen it when I've had the lung function test.

ALI: Spirometry?

CHERYL: What's that?

ALI: Where you blow into this machine and they have you breathe in different ways. They try to capture how your lungs are functioning.

CHERYL: Oh yeah, so the first time, when I was at Temple, I used it. But I recently had it in July at the pulmonologist, so this time I got to sit down and watch the graph.

ALI: What did you learn?

CHERYL: I think being able to see the graph and I'm trying to reach the points or whatever point that is considered going good or whatever, I feel like that kind of messed with my own judgment of how my lungs are doing. I'm trying to reach whatever point that is the okay level instead of really seeing how my lungs are doing. So I don't know about other people, but for me, just being able to see—okay, I'm trying to get to this point but it's not my normal breathing.

ALI: But the app *does* get at your everyday breathing. Do you like the app? Do you find the app useful?

CHERYL: Yeah, sometimes it's annoying. But I can like check in real quick and I know if I'm like not having the best day as far as breathing, then I get reminders and suggestions. Do I use them? Depends on what it is. It's probably things that I already know. But you can adjust the settings. But you have to contact Blue Cross to change, like, your daily habits. So it's based off of me and my daily habits as far as how active I am and stuff like that. So if that changes, the bases change. I don't think it's something I can do myself. I have to contact them to change it, and that's annoying. It's convenient because it's on my phone, but—

ALI: But you don't actually use their tips.

CHERYL: A lot of them I already know what I should be doing. So if I know my lungs are constricted or whatever, I know I should be taking the albuterol. So, I don't need you to tell me that.

ALI: Are there things that you know you should do that you don't do?

CHERYL: Yeah. So now I just . . . There was a long time that I wasn't carrying a rescue inhaler. Now I'm definitely trying to be more conscious of it. But I guess it took other things to happen before I saw like, oh, I should really carry this. Like, more recently, with food allergies. Eating things and having reactions.

Cheryl's comments highlight two disjunctions between knowledge and care. First, note the distance between Cheryl's perception of her breathing and the representation of Cheryl's breathing produced by either the spirometer or the Care Cam app. Part of the work that asthma care apps aim to do is bring patient perceptions of disease in line with clinical assessment metrics, like peak flow readings. Second, while Cheryl was now receiving basic disease management tips from an app, she had yet to receive basic treatment tools, including an asthma action plan and a peak flow meter, from her health care provider. She might have received these tools when she was first diagnosed as a child, or later as a teen, when she began taking on more responsibility for her health care, but her health care providers had not asked about her use of either in a number of years. Such gaps between illness experience and treatment regimen are produced by specific configurations of chronic care infrastructures, especially the doctor–patient interaction. Clinical visits establish the terms of diagnosis and treatment, and doctors can help establish care continuity. But even with regular access to health insurance, Cheryl seemed to be lacking continuity in care.

Like many of the breathers discussed in earlier chapters, Cheryl defined "controlled asthma" as the absence of embodied symptoms. She did not think in terms of clinical asthma control or future risk. Cheryl's definition of control related specifically to how her lungs felt to her. She could describe the scary feeling of not being able to breathe, but the graph of her lung function threw her off. The Care Cam app that Cheryl received from her insurance company, however, worked to capture both clinical readings—peak flow readings—and self-perception. It gave Cheryl the option of entering peak flow readings, but it also asked her to rank and characterize her breathing on a numeric scale based on her own sense of her breathing body. Cheryl found this daily tracking feature useful. She liked having a day-to-day record of how she was feeling. In this sense, the Care Cam app gave asthmatic attunement a digital structure and archived it.[20] The app, provided by an insurance company, is designed to cultivate daily awareness and prompt self-control behaviors that manage body and environment and, presumably, reduce health care spending. Mobile health apps work through consistent collection of behavioral, biological, and subjective data, which can be translated into analytics that present cause-and-effect relationships in the form of user trends or can be paired with health education that points users to different actions. Cheryl, however, did not find this information terribly useful, as it mainly replicated things she had already been told. It did not add anything "new."

A key aim of many digital health projects is to regularize and reinforce health maintenance activities, such as taking peak flow readings and tracking how a patient feels. In Cheryl's case, however, the app's ability to provide rhythmic, continuous care depended on the doctor–patient relationship, which seemed somewhat lacking. For the app to structure her care, Cheryl needed to have the right care apparatus and guidance from a medical provider. Without a peak flow meter or a current asthma action plan, Cheryl could not use the app effectively. The app's ability to carry out its functions depended on the quality of the chronic care infrastructure. An asthma care app can improve a patient's care only if the patient has access to medical care—to say nothing of *good* medical care.[21]

In our conversation, Cheryl mentioned some of the hoops in the health care system she had to jump through in search of medical care prior to the passage of the ACA. She described bouncing back and forth between insurance providers and medical centers as her mother's health insurance coverage changed, and when Cheryl changed schools or jobs. Her story highlights how breathers are embedded within and dependent on health care services, which are uneven, complex, and experienced differently over time and place. Cheryl's story offers a snapshot of the emergent and complex qualities of the U.S. health care system. Disease management apps enter into and exist within the system's complex care infrastructures. While these technologies promise to improve care by gathering data that can help patients better understand their disease, track treatment, and communicate with health care providers, none of these outcomes were met in Cheryl's experience.

Six months after my first interview with Cheryl, I asked her for a follow-up interview to talk more about Care Cam. I wanted to analyze its design as I had analyzed those of other asthma care apps. We set a meeting time, but then she e-mailed to tell me that Care Cam was gone—it was no longer on her phone. Her health insurance company's app was still there, but Care Cam was nowhere to be found. There was no trace of it on her phone or on the Blue Cross website. Although Cheryl used the app consistently when she first downloaded it, after a few months her use gradually decreased. By the time we spoke, she had not used the app in several months. This is a common pattern of use that has been documented in studies that have looked at various kinds of apps.[22]

After various internet searches, the two of us realized that Care Cam had morphed into a different app called The Voyage, no longer associated with Blue Cross. "Apparently my insurance isn't partnered with the company anymore since there is no trace of the app on their website, which seems weird. I downloaded [The Voyage] to see if it's the same. Some of the questions are, but the app itself is really annoying and intrusive! There's no way I would continue using it," Cheryl told me. She felt that the new app requested too much personal information. I pointed out to her that the original Care Cam used her insurance ID number, which may have pulled in patient information. This gave her pause. The way the app had been recommended to her made it appear as if Care Cam was associated with Blue Cross. Now that it was clear that a third-party company owned the app, Cheryl was uncomfortable with using it. And she had no idea what kind of access either company had to her medical records.

Over the eight-year span of this project, I have documented notable changes in both the design and the features of personal health technologies as well as in their relationships to insurance companies and large health care organizations. Hospitals, for instance, encourage their patients to use apps to reduce the costs of care. It should be no surprise that the logic of asthma control, discussed in chapter 2, rules these developments, or that health maintenance organizations, for example, have begun offering such apps to clients. It was not clear in 2010, however, that asthma care apps would develop in this way. In fact, in 2010, app developers believed that it was by virtue of GPS that smartphones would "revolutionize" asthma care through public health research, rather than through a logic of asthma control anchored in medication adherence.

The Science of Asthma Care Apps

While the vast majority of the apps profiled thus far were developed by individuals unaffiliated with health care organizations or by teams of developers situated within clinics, hospitals, or insurance companies, researchers represent another group of app users, albeit a group that has entered the fray more slowly.

In March 2015, Apple announced the release of ResearchKit, an open-source software framework that would "revolutionize medical studies" by helping doctors and scientists "gather data more frequently and more accurately from participants."[23] Apple additionally claimed that ResearchKit would bridge the gap between research and care. In a promotional video posted on Apple's ResearchKit website, ResearchKit developers, researchers, and patients describe how these new apps have changed the way they interface with disease. "ResearchKit has clearly transformed research. More importantly, it's laid the foundation to transform care," says Dr. Ray Dorsey of the University of Rochester, who has used ResearchKit's mPower app to study Parkinson's disease. Divya Nag, an Apple representative, declares, "This is no longer just about research. People are using apps to learn about themselves in a way that they couldn't before to create a better life for themselves in terms of their own health." Patients with epilepsy and Parkinson's disease describe how daily assessments help them learn about the contours of their own individual disease. Their stories emphasize that thanks to good design and user data, care is becoming more personalized. The scientists featured in the video, meanwhile, underscore that ResearchKit gives them larger numbers of research participants than they have ever had access to before.[24]

At the launch for ResearchKit, Apple also announced the release of five apps, each focusing on a different disease condition, developed by partner organizations during the platform's development phase. One of these apps, the Asthma Health Application (AHA), was developed by a team from Mount Sinai's Icahn School of Medicine. As described by its developers on the project website, AHA "is a personalized tool that helps you to gain greater insight into your asthma, avoid triggers, adhere to treatment plans, and take charge of your health." The description continues:

> The Asthma Health app helps you to track your asthma symptoms, allows you to review trends, gives you feedback on your progress, and provides personalized reminders to take your prescribed medications. The Asthma Health app has even added new features that allow you to share information collected on the app with your doctor.
>
> We aim to help patients experience fewer asthma-related limitations and less distress—with better symptom control, fewer unexpected medical visits, and improved quality of life.[25]

Although this description resembles those of other asthma care apps, the fact that AHA is built on the ResearchKit platform increases its utility for medical research. Like Propeller, AHA leverages smartphone data in new ways to produce insights on the asthma epidemic, its relation to the environment, and disease management practices. The question remains, however, whether the data are good for science.

In the study reported in the first peer-reviewed article published on AHA, the researchers focused on care outcomes as well as on the methodological issues involved in using mobile apps for health research.[26] Although AHA was downloaded almost 50,000 times in the first six months of its release, only 8,524 users—fewer than 1 in 5—completed the electronic consent process. An additional 1,000 potential users failed to complete the e-mail confirmation necessary to enroll in the study. The cohort was, however, comparable with the general U.S. asthma population as indicated by CDC asthma surveillance data, and the patient-reported outcomes were structured similarly to those in traditional epidemiological studies. These two important dimensions put the AHA study on par with other public health research. The researchers also found that the user-reported asthma triggers correlated with externally validated environmental events, based on data reported by federal air monitors and weather stations. In terms of care outcomes, user self-reports indicated that the app helped with disease management and reduced users' activity limitations. Among users who stuck with AHA for a six-month period, the data also indicated a significant increase in asthma control (according to GINA standards). In concluding their article, the researchers describe the results as encouraging but limited, noting that "validating the clinical impact of AHA usage warrants rigorous future clinical trials."[27]

Participant retention posed a significant challenge in this study. At the six-month mark, only a very small subset of the initial enrollment group (175 participants) completed the six-month survey. Given that testing the potential of app-based platforms like ResearchKit for use in conducting public health research was part of the point of the project, the researchers found this level of attrition informative. They note in their report that such a steep decline in user participation parallels the declines found in many other digital use cases, a situation that they characterize as "speak[ing] to the hardwired biopsychosocial tendencies of users." If the goal of mobile health studies is the collection of longitudinal data, they observe, then "the creators of these tools must understand users' psychosocial-behavioral needs and predilections to keep them continually engaged."[28] Even aside from the issue of whether the data collected by ResearchKit and similar apps are reliable, the first hurdle seems to be getting people to use care apps consistently over time. The value of the apps, in other words, is data dependent.

To help promote the project, AHA investigators also curated participant testimonials (posted on the project website) and created a map of participant distribution across the lower forty-eight U.S. states.[29] The Asthma Health Map shows the number and location of participants by state, as well as their reported triggers. These include strong smells in Nebraska and Texas, and poor air quality in Nevada, Alabama, and Michigan. Cold air has been reported as a trigger in Iowa, Kansas, Minnesota, and New Hampshire, and mold in Washington, Minnesota, Mississippi, and Pennsylvania. Exercise, cats and dogs, stress, weather changes, dust, pollen, and smoking are other reported triggers. Snippets of testimonials line the edges of the map, documenting participants' satisfaction with AHA (the full testimonials are available on the website's "Participant Stories" page). "I used to think my asthma was just symptoms related to allergies," says Sharon A. of Camarillo, California. She credits AHA with giving her a much richer picture of her disease. She explains that she went to see an allergist after her asthma and allergies started bothering her more, at which point she downloaded the app. She used it daily for eight months:

One of the main things the Asthma App has done for me is that it has made me aware of how predictable my asthma is. I've found that the consistency of the questions asked in the app has made me much more aware of how asthma is impacting my daily life. I now know how important it is for me to take my medications. I also really like the articles that pop up. They constantly keep me up to date on the latest asthma-related news.

. . . It's great and doesn't take a lot of time out of my day. I would often forget to take my medications, but the reminders on the app have really helped me remember. I also feel that the app is very responsive and it holds me accountable for my asthma.[30]

The testimonials narrate a broad range of care app benefits. Sharon likes AHA's consistency and structure, for example, and believes it helps her stay on top of managing her disease. The rhythmic care infrastructure cultivates awareness and has shown Sharon that her asthma is actually predictable. Sharon (and a number of other participants) also values the patient education aspects of AHA, including its updates about asthma research and news. Indeed, patient education seemed to be one of AHA's core goals, a move to compensate for an overburdened health care system and limitations in doctor–patient care dynamics.

Of the nine participants profiled on the website, three mention the value of contributing to asthma research in their testimonials. Nicholas H. of Seattle, Washington, is impressed with the structure and clarity of AHA: "It was very clear to me who was doing the research, why the research was being done, and how the data will be used and shared." Nicholas comments specifically on the utility of tracking peak flow readings, which he has found to be the most useful feature of the app. He is also happy to be able to see his own data, which might otherwise be viewable only by researchers: "I find it rewarding to be part of a research study that is the new model of the future—not in the traditional, old-school approach where we are not able to view our own data." Danielle T. of Colorado Springs, Colorado, similarly joined the study to help advance asthma science—to the point that she did not think that enrolling in the study might change her own view of and relationship to asthma care. Her testimonial presents AHA as a tool to improve her disease management:

"The app has also provided unexpected personal benefits that have made a positive impact on my overall health and wellbeing." When Danielle meets with her doctor she is now able to say, with confidence and data: "I'm having these symptoms, at this frequency. Doctor, should we change my medicine dose?" Danielle says her doctor has been very receptive and impressed with the heightened level of self-knowledge that she now has. "I am now much more actively involved in my healthcare and I'm pleased that I was able to partner with my doctor to create my Asthma Plan."

Michael K. of Evansville, Indiana, echoes Danielle's comment about how AHA has strengthened the doctor–patient relationship and says that the app helps him get more out of his appointments. "I also find the charts on doctor dashboard very handy for my physician. I only see him every three months, but with the app, I can gauge my asthma daily and answer my doctor's questions more accurately." Michael's comments point to AHA's value for both public health and self-care. "Not many people understand how fast-growing asthma is and how much it hinders daily activity," he says, but AHA has provided him with new knowledge of the disease. Nor is Michael alone in referring to how his increased self-knowledge has improved his interactions with his medical team. AHA's design, with its "doctor dashboard," seems to facilitate support for treatment providers.

Michael's favorite feature on the app, however, is "the environmental data." In his testimonial, he says, "I'm really affected by pollen and knowing the air quality helps me figure out what kind of day I will have." Understanding the relationships among disease, symptoms, and environment is something mentioned in many of the AHA participant testimonials. This was something that the principal investigators at Mount Sinai tracked as well. In media reports and the peer-reviewed article on their findings, the researchers highlighted the wildfires in Washington State in the summer of 2015 as an event that allowed them to detect and correlate "a marked increase in our study participants' daily asthma symptoms . . . with real-time fine particulate matter (Environmental Protection Agency air quality logs PM 2.5) levels in regions affected by wildfires during those corresponding time periods."[31] The location-specific user data gathered by AHA, coupled with environmental data, showed a strong correlation between wildfires and asthma symptoms.

The AHA researchers found the wildfires useful as an extreme event that allowed them to evaluate the validity of the app's data. But for people with asthma, using an app to track their symptoms along with changing environmental conditions offers a new, mediated way to practice attunement. AHA users check in with environmental features daily, as a rhythmic intervention to help prepare for their day.[32] In her AHA testimonial, Michelle S. of Queens, New York, writes, "I also use the app to analyze air quality. For example, when I travel, I track the difference between the clean air of upstate New York and the more polluted air of New York

City, and look for correlations to my asthma condition." Another user, Amanda H. of Dallas, Texas, says, "I like that it displays the local air quality and provides a particle count." She notes that tracking her asthma with the app "brought up ideas about my triggers that I had never thought of before." Amanda had recently been diagnosed with exercise-induced asthma, but a bout of pneumonia had escalated the disease. At first, she had a hard time distinguishing between her asthma and other forms of disordered breathing, but AHA helped her connect her symptoms to the environment in new ways.

Sourcing Environmental Health Data

ResearchKit is a potent example of how smartphone apps can transform medical research by translating patient care into data through a greater number of registers and scales than ever before. Both the Propeller app and AHA show how large-scale mobile asthma apps have the potential to connect individual symptoms—that is, data involving place and time—to environmental data. The potential for gathering environmental data has attracted the attention of nearly every developer involved in mobile asthma apps. Clinical practitioners, meanwhile, emphasize the use of apps to increase their patients' adherence to their treatment regimens, first and foremost. While some developers and company representatives convey that all pillars of care are important for asthma control, others lean toward treatment adherence. Again, it matters where the app and its stakeholders are situated.

Steve, the app developer whose three-year-old son had asthma, stated that he wanted to integrate environmental data into Asthma Edge:

> That is one of the things on my big ideas list, is to find a public weather source that I can use to either say, if this is your location, this is your pollen count today. Or something like that. Or in a more predictive way—say, the pollen count is going to be X tomorrow, be prepared. Be aware of your symptoms or something like that. So it doesn't do it yet, but like I said, this matters to me because one of the triggers for my son is allergies, so that kind of information would be helpful. Living where we do, I don't listen to the weather forecast every day because it doesn't change day to day that much. So something that tells me proactively would be good.

Steve wanted to be preemptive, proactive, and preventive about his son's asthma, and he thought others would also want to be alerted to changing environmental conditions that could trigger symptoms. Unfortunately for Steve's app, Steve came to this realization later than other developers.

Considered next to Propeller, AHA, or Asthma Ally (which features daily atmospheric conditions right on the dashboard), Asthma Edge lacks many of the locational features that emerging asthma care apps boast. Steve, of course, works alone, whereas AHA is supported by Mount Sinai, and Propeller Health has a long list of corporate partners.

Bill, an app development team member for a health management organization who worked on the user interface for his company's asthma app, echoed Steve's vision. In his mind, the app could serve as a kind of warning system: "The idea was, maybe we provide a warning system for people who live in a certain area, that all of this ozone is going up, you can get a text message to say, listen, in your area—because we know where all these numbers are and where people are, because everything is GPS now." Gene, a marketing expert at a tech start-up that had developed another of the asthma care apps I surveyed, said something similar. He suggested that push notifications could preemptively alert users to atmospheric conditions that might make it more difficult to breathe:

> Ultimately the goal is to have a database of information on asthma
> practice and on asthma care and multiple sensor systems feeding data
> into that database and then based upon that database, we hope to
> apply an algorithm to be able to predict increasing risk to the patient.
> So we know that the behavior of an asthmatic is important, but we also
> know it's not all the time the behavior, there may be external stimuli,
> environmental stimuli. So one of the things that the smartphone allows
> us to do, is to use the GPS, and that looks out at the environment and
> collects information about not only the person's location, but what is the
> environment he's in? Is there poor air quality at this time? Is the pollen
> count up? And then collectively, in a community way, we can look and
> say, by the way, ten to twenty asthmatics in your neighborhood have
> just taken their rescue inhalers. And you should be aware.

Gene's vision of environmental app notifications goes well beyond the verified environmental data that AHA uses to validate user-entered data. Because the emphasis is on user-driven information rather than on public health research, notifications could draw on local, crowdsourced data from other app users' symptom and exposure data. At the time of this writing, no asthma care apps use this kind of real-time, crowdsourced data, and— Gene's comments notwithstanding—it is not clear that any will go in this direction. Nonetheless, Gene's vision of how databases and algorithms could be used for a kind of collective, public care for asthma is part of an emerging technoscientific imaginary that may be pushing innovation in app design across the field.

While almost every developer I spoke with expressed intellectual curiosity about the potential of connecting environmental data to patient data, not everyone saw environmental information as useful for patient care. Some interlocutors, particularly those with clinical backgrounds, insisted that the potential of apps to increase adherence to prescribed asthma medications could do more for public health than providing asthma sufferers with information on pollen counts, air quality, or the weather. According to these physicians, patients who are taking their medications as prescribed—that is, those with well-controlled asthma—should not be adversely affected by routine environmental events. The comments of Bill, a development team member at a state-level health management organization, are representative of this point of view:

> It is certainly very good information to know from a population health standpoint, but it would be something that would be difficult for an individual to act upon. Whereas if somebody is not taking their meds, then that needs to be addressed immediately and could be addressed immediately using our tool. We have been focusing more on the behavior components and things that we can correct to get the user back on the adherence track. There might be additional improvements available from a population health standpoint, but ours is really more on an individual patient, individual transaction basis.

Mark, another member of the same HMO development team, stated that the nature of environmental risk exceeds the realm of individual agency. People with asthma cannot control atmospheric pressure or air quality, but they can adhere to their treatment regimens. They can take responsibility for taking their medications. This perspective holds that the public health problems caused by air pollution and high pollen counts are best addressed through medication regimens that provide breathers with biochemical protection from a deteriorating environment. On an individual basis, patients who routinely take their medications are less likely to miss school or work because of complications from asthma. Here, it is important to keep in mind that the particular app being developed by the HMO team was primarily for use by Medicaid recipients. The app's explicit focus was to improve clients' overall health to reduce public health expenditures in the form of emergency room visits and hospitalizations, and to increase productivity and educational outcomes by minimizing work and school absences.

Dr. Wilson helped to develop an app that was not explicitly aimed at increasing adherence, but he nevertheless suggested that this might be an appropriate role for asthma care apps. When I asked him if he thought air quality data and alerts would be useful for his patients, he was dismissive: "That is not asking the right question. [We should be] asking a question like why are the asthma rates so high and why is adherence so low? What can we do about that? We know that that is causing the problem, the majority of the problem is by nonadherence and not proper management. So what can we do about that?" Wilson thought it would be more fruitful to investigate why people are not taking their medications and what barriers they face in adhering to treatment.

At the time of this writing, almost all mobile asthma apps, even those that draw on environmental data, focus on adherence. Perhaps this is not surprising given that most asthma care apps are now being developed with backing from insurance companies, inhaler manufacturers, and major hospital systems. Nevertheless, many individual developers I spoke with offered a range of perspectives on how mobile asthma apps might transform patient care. Gene articulated an overarching goal for an effective app that captures well the foundational values of all asthma care apps, regardless of their mix of care logics or their dominant aims:

> The app will raise a dialogue. In reality, a well-controlled asthmatic doesn't think he's an asthmatic. That is the psychology of asthma that makes it such a unique disease. Because when you are well controlled, you are as normal as the next girl. Or the next guy. You have no concept of being asthmatic. It's completely out of mind. This will serve as a reminder and it would be a negative reminder maybe in your mentality, but also it would raise the issue—I'm an asthmatic.

Gene's view reifies the emphasis on the asthmatic and knowledge of the self. In order for there to be data to work with—for there to be data that can care in the first place—breathers need to become aware of their disease in ways that call for certain kinds of care. Digital therapeutics—a term that refers to apps that are designed to treat disease by modifying patient behavior—requires patients who can be plugged into existing and emerging health care systems.[33]

As one of the very first mobile asthma apps, and certainly the most widely publicized, Propeller was quick to receive attention, praise, and monetary investment.[34] Over the subsequent nine years, the app won countless awards, was the subject of spotlight presentations at conferences and events, and anchored multiple studies on asthma treatment outcomes.[35] Its proponents have raised more than fifteen million dollars to support the project, and Propeller Health has developed civic partnerships to facilitate data collection for proof of concept.[36] With the change in name in September

2013, Propeller Health's branding shifted from a focus on collecting data for asthma research to improving clinical outcomes for a broader palette of respiratory diseases, including chronic obstructive pulmonary disease.[37] A new promotional video titled *Live Your Life without Limits* paints a remarkably different picture from that presented in the 2010 video described at the beginning of this chapter. The more recent video begins with an animated view of a factory spewing smoke into the surrounding trees. The scene then morphs into a ball and chain attached to a young woman's ankle:

> If you have asthma or COPD, managing your disease can take over your life. You have to constantly remember when to take your medications and manually keep track of your symptoms. You even wind up avoiding certain activities out of fear that they'll trigger an attack. Propeller makes managing asthma and COPD easier than ever. It gives you the confidence to live the life that you want to live. The Propeller sensor attaches to your inhalers and records when, where, and why you have symptoms. So you can prevent attacks before they happen. Your doctor can see how you're doing as well, allowing them to tailor the treatment plan that's right for you. Users have up to 70 percent fewer attacks and up to 50 percent more symptom-free days. So instead of worrying about what might cause an attack, you can take control of your life and do the things you love to do. Live your life without limits. Propeller: Learn more today.[38]

Gone are snapshots of neighborhood maps showing where people are using rescue inhalers. The collective view of disordered breathing amid environmental hot spots, which were shown through satellite images in the first video, has been replaced by doctor–patient interaction. After showing how the sensor fits onto a rescue inhaler, the video cuts to a symptom log with time and date information. A happy-looking doctor jumps into view and reviews the same woman's health data alongside Propeller's outcome statistics. The doctor then hands the woman an inhaler. By the end of the video, the woman is able to remove her ball and chain to join her friends playing baseball. Whereas the 2010 Propeller Health video ends with a promise to transform asthma research to improve public health outcomes, the 2016 video focuses on how users can "take control of life" and live "without limits."

There are certainly overlaps between the videos—both leverage the promise of data, and the 2016 video opens with a picture of air pollution. Nevertheless, the later video minimizes the potential of technology to address a public health crisis in favor of shoring up individualized asthma control. Instead of the hopeful tone of the original, which suggests that patients, researchers, and the broader public might learn more about asthma and the asthma epidemic from the data gathered by the app, the newer video promises that Propeller will help individuals avoid stress and reclaim their lives through better disease management.

These promotional videos, however, fail to highlight the company's growing public health research. CEO David Van Sickle and his extensive network of collaborators, which includes municipalities, tech firms, pharmaceutical companies, and other researchers, have published nearly a dozen peer-reviewed articles in public health journals based on Propeller. In a 2017 article published in *Environmental Health Perspectives*, Jason G. Su and his coauthors (one of whom is David Van Sickle) lay out an impressive picture of how the researchers paired data passively collected through the Propeller sensor with data on common environmental triggers and factors from the built environment. Using federal data sets, the study

> confirmed that it is feasible to use data collected by the inhaler sensors to investigate the relationships among asthma rescue inhaler use, environmental triggers, and built environment factors. Several environmental triggers were found to be associated with increased inhaler use, such as AQI, PM_{10}, weed pollen, and mold. Conversely, tree cover demonstrated protective effects. The lessons learned from this feasibility study have informed the design of the expanded study currently underway in Louisville, and will help investigate these associations further. The application of these new technologies has the potential to improve our understanding of asthma, both for clinical disease management and public health.[39]

The idea that app developers must choose between promoting clinical disease management and advancing public health science is false. An app can do both, as Propeller has demonstrated. Its ability to do both, however, is based on an element of chronic care infrastructure that sets it apart from all other asthma care apps: passive data collection.

Propeller remains the only asthma care app that uses a device in addition to a smartphone. The GPS sensor that is attached to the user's rescue inhaler tracks medication use automatically, both through time and in space. The system does not depend on manual entry, a problem identified by the AHA team at Mount Sinai, whose study had poor rates of user retention, which in turn produced a steep drop-off in longitudinal data. (This problem is not unique to mobile asthma apps—it plagues all clinical and public health studies.) Of course, the very element that sets Propeller apart has attracted criticism. The GPS sensor, critics told me, is something users have to obtain and manage, at extra cost. But in practice, once users have attached the sensors to their inhalers, Propeller requires very little user effort or even awareness. User data generated automatically by the smart inhaler go directly to Propeller's information systems, at which point they are analyzed and kicked back out to users in the form of notifications and data visualizations. A recent article on lessons the company learned in its first decade notes that Propeller Health's CTO Greg Tracy has observed that the most important thing was not to try to change patients' habits or lives—the technology had to fit seamlessly into existing lifestyles.[40] This is a message that seems to be the opposite of what many asthma care apps and mobile health platforms, with their breathless emphasis on behavioral change, hope to achieve.

Propeller Health has not built this infrastructure alone. The company's website notes that Propeller Health is "delivering improved outcomes to over thirty large healthcare systems, integrated delivery networks, pharmacy benefit mangers, and self-insured employers." As of the time of this writing, the company has received eight FDA approvals for sensors to be used on different inhalers.[41] The pharmaceutical industry is enthusiastic about Propeller Health's potential to transform asthma care. Following FDA approval for a Propeller attachment to a GlaxoSmithKline inhaler in 2016, Dave Allen, GSK's head of respiratory research and development, remarked:

> While it is still in the early stages of development, the emerging field of digital healthcare holds great promise for respiratory medicine. The approval of the Propeller platform for use with the Ellipta inhaler will help us understand how patients interact with the Ellipta inhaler accurately and in real-time. By exploring the benefits of sensor technology in this way, we hope to gain valuable insights into usage patterns with the ultimate goal of driving improvements in patient care while reducing the complexity and cost of clinical trials.[42]

This relationship between GlaxoSmithKline and Propeller Health signals the rise of digital therapeutics, yes, but also an approach that offers a kind of mobile health platform that is different from the wellness or fitness apps that have received so much attention in the medical technology world. Rather than asking patients to track their disease in place, Propeller gathers data from the users' already existing care infrastructure: the inhaler. As technologies that support medical treatment, digital therapeutics are often backed by pharmaceutical or insurance companies. With so many layers of interest and investment, it will be interesting to see how these different modes of digital health care delivery play out in asthma care. No doubt patient-consumers will experience these modes in various ways, depending on the configuration of their relationships to chronic care infrastructures, including access to insurance and continuity of care. And it will also be worth observing how emerging asthma care apps call attention to local and global air pollution in more nuanced ways, as Propeller and AHA are striving to do, making more robust connections between respiratory health and environmental exposures.

CHAPTER FIVE

Public Health Carescapes for Climate Change

In the United States, asthma care has been directed primarily at individual breathers. Both pharmaceutical treatments and mobile asthma apps, for example, work on an individual basis. Even when asthma apps are designed with the care team in mind, they focus on changing the behavior of the person with asthma. The Buteyko breathing technique is also meant for individual sufferers, who can learn to shift their respiratory rhythms with a routine breath control practice. While these modes of asthma care do involve communities of practice, such as the community of Buteyko breathing educators and the care networks of researchers and doctors who are drawn in by app infrastructure, none of these approaches constitute interventions in public health. Their advocates may hope for broad impact— for every person diagnosed with asthma to receive breathing lessons when prescribed an inhaler, for instance, or for app users' crowdsourced care data to provide better insight into air pollution hot spots—but none of these modes of care can be considered public health interventions as they stand. Yet the asthma epidemic *is* a public health issue, and the disease disproportionately affects individuals, families, and communities living in low-income urban areas, where poverty, environmental racism, and inadequate housing conditions not only produce disordered breathing but also make caring for it particularly difficult.[1]

Philadelphia is a city that has long struggled with high asthma prevalence rates and poor control among those diagnosed. According to the Pennsylvania Department of Health, Philadelphia County's three-year asthma prevalence rate for the period 2011–13 was 19 percent, more than double the national average of 7.6 percent. Childhood prevalence rates were also nearly three times the national average for childhood asthma, with nearly one in four children in Philadelphia living with an asthma diagnosis.[2] According to the Philadelphia Department of Public Health's (PDPH) 2014 Community Health Assessment, child asthma hospitalization rates more than doubled from 2000 to 2010, with the highest rates recorded among black children and children of all races living in the River Wards, a city planning district that borders the I-95 corridor and hosts some of the highest concentrations of industry in the city.[3] Decades of research on asthma in Philadelphia poignantly show that poverty, aging housing stock, and poor air quality make the city unbreathable for its most vulnerable citizens.[4]

Across the city, formal networks of organizations and looser groups of affiliates provide programming to address the asthma epidemic as a public health crisis. A number of these programs focus on children and operate through the School District of Philadelphia; others operate through local hospitals. While these two kinds of institutions, schools and hospitals, have been at the forefront of public health interventions for asthma since the epidemic began in the 1980s, grassroots movements and environmental justice organizations have also played a role in some U.S. cities. In Philadelphia, three such initiatives have emerged in recent years to combat the city's asthma epidemic. In the Healthy Rowhouse Project, a coalition of organizations work to address asthma and other environmental health issues, including childhood lead exposure, by confronting the city's aging and dilapidated housing stock. A second movement centers on Philly Thrive, a grassroots coalition formed to protest the creation of a proposed "energy hub" that would expand an oil and gas refinery in Philadelphia's already heavily polluted Southwest district.[5] The third initiative, the focus of this chapter, is the Climate, Health, and Home project, a workshop series that brought together innovative climate change education, social scientific expertise, and public health service provision. The broad network of organizations, programs, and resources working to address the Philadelphia asthma epidemic can be characterized as a *carescape*, a place-based landscape of services and relationships knit together by macro-level factors that include not only federal and state policies, economic conditions, new technologies, and health delivery systems but also the specific needs of the population.[6]

The Climate, Health, and Home project, with which I was involved, differed from the existing initiatives in Philadelphia's carescape by embracing an orientation toward preparing for future environmental and infrastructural threats—specifically, the threats of climate change. A significant portion of the project focused on community education and outreach about the relationship between climate change and health. Workshops offered tips for increasing energy efficiency in homes, for instance, and addressed the specific vulnerabilities of senior citizens to hot weather. By working through the existing asthma carescape, which included the Philadelphia Department of Public Health and local "healthy homes" programs, Climate, Health, and Home aimed to bring new forms of expertise and services to Philadelphia communities burdened by asthma while at the same time expanding the range of ways in which the city could address a looming public health crisis. The project also leveraged funding for climate change education and drew on federal publications to communicate the health impacts of climate change. This reinforced the message that asthma is an environmental health disease intimately shaped by ecology, infrastructure, and atmospheric conditions.

In this chapter, I describe how the Climate, Health, and Home workshop series addressed asthma care by framing the epidemic as a climate change issue. In so doing, the project brought together public and private tactics and resources that could be used by Philadelphia's most vulnerable citizens. I also reflect on my own involvement with the project to explore how research and public health collaboration carries with it a politics of care.[7]

Staying Cool in a Changing Climate

"Has anyone experienced climate change, here in Philadelphia?" I asked the packed room. "Any of the conditions you just mentioned?" Although we had started the workshop fifteen minutes late, I wanted to make sure people shared their personal experiences as much as possible.

"Well, it's hotter," a woman in the middle of the room exclaimed. "It's so hot I don't even want to move around my house. And I have air-conditioning!"[8] Across the room people nodded in agreement, and some chimed in with various affirmations. "The weather is just funny," another woman spoke up. "You can experience four seasons in one day. You don't know what to expect."

"Asthma and allergies are at an all-time high. Things are out of whack," said a man at the front of the room. "I don't even have asthma and I have a hard time breathing around Center City, with all the smells and the cars. I never used to have this problem." Other people offered their own experiences in response. A handful of the workshop participants related that they had developed asthma and allergies as adults. A man in the back said it felt like the city had more mold, which was one of his asthma triggers. I let the room bubble for a few more minutes as people took turns sharing their experiences with weather, health, and the built environment.

"Okay, so it sounds like you all have intimate experiences with Philadelphia's environment and the changes under way," I said as I switched out my PowerPoint presentation and loaded the next. "Our first presenter is Russ Zerbo from Clean Air Council. Russ is going to give some more information about the mechanisms of climate change. He's also going to show you some local environmental data, and talk more about what climate change will look like in Philadelphia in the years to come." As I sat down to the side as Russ took the floor, I reflected on how often participants brought up asthma, even if we did not. Perhaps I should not have found this surprising. According to the Asthma and Allergy Foundation of America, Philadelphia ranks third among the most difficult cities in the United States to live in with asthma.[9]

The group of seniors participating in the workshop, titled "Staying Cool in a Changing Climate," were packed into one of the classrooms at the new South Philadelphia branch of the Free Library of Philadelphia, the city's public library system. The workshop was designed to raise awareness among senior citizens of the health impacts of heat waves, or what the Philadelphia Department of Public Health had started referring to as "heat health emergencies." In Philadelphia, a heat health emergency is declared when the heat index (temperature plus humidity) crests 105 degrees for two consecutive days. The declaration activates a number of city services, such as cooling centers, additional resources for people experiencing homelessness, and the Philadelphia Corporation for Aging's Heatline, a telephone service that provides information specific to heat waves and city resources. The city halts utility shutoffs during a heat health emergency, and PDPH launches a mobile unit to make home visits, thus extending health care access to those unable to travel safely during a heat wave. Information about the services available during a heat health emergency is posted on a web page accessible through the Office of Emergency Management, which also provides a link to an interactive city resource map that shows the locations of cooling centers and "spraygrounds."[10] One of the aims of the workshop was to make sure that senior citizens had access to this information whether or not they had access to a computer.

PDPH and other Climate, Health, and Home project partners had identified heat health emergencies as a critical and pressing topic to address. More than just heat, warm weather produces favorable conditions for some types of air pollution, like ground-level ozone, which can trigger asthma symptoms for some people. And indeed, the day after this workshop was held, the Pennsylvania Department of Environmental Protection declared a "Code Orange Air Quality Action Day" as temperatures approached 100 degrees.[11] A Code Orange day is one in which air pollution levels reach the rating of "unhealthy for sensitive groups" according to the U.S. Environmental Protection Agency's Air Quality Index (AQI).

The AQI represents the cumulative air pollution level (for all six criteria pollutants regulated by the Clean Air Act) in a geographic area. In 2016, Philadelphia County had nine Code Orange days based on the AQI value for total city air pollution.[12] Such air quality action days are expected to increase in frequency with climate change, a trend that will have dramatic consequences for public health, and particularly for vulnerable populations, including children, the elderly, and people with respiratory disorders.

"Who can tell us what a cooling center is?" Teija Corse, the PDPH workshop facilitator, asked the group. No one answered. People seemed to be thinking about the question. Not missing a beat, Teija launched into a description: "Well, you're in a designated cooling center right now. Cooling centers are air-conditioned spaces that are open to the public during heat waves. They are usually recreational centers, public libraries, or community centers. Always call the city's Heatline or 311 to find out which ones have been activated, though." Once she explained the term, the participants immediately recognized the service; a few offered that they had used cooling centers during past heat health emergencies. No one had known the official term *cooling center,* however. Since part of the project goal was to get a sense of what Philadelphians knew about climate change, its health risks, and related city services, this was useful information. Based on workshops run over the previous three summers, we knew that *cooling centers* was not a term used widely in West Philadelphia and the River Wards, the communities where we were doing outreach. This year, we had purposely scheduled all three workshops at designated city cooling centers: the West Philadelphia Senior Community Center and the South Philadelphia and McPherson (Kensington) branches of the Free Library. Our hope was that workshop participants would later remember these sites as places where they could take refuge during heat health emergencies.

Teija went on to describe the possible health hazards of heat waves, including dehydration, heatstroke, and, of course, respiratory symptoms like asthma attacks. Extreme heat events can exacerbate existing medical conditions and alter how the body processes medical treatments such as pharmaceuticals. This message was particularly important to convey to seniors, who are more likely than those who are younger to be living with chronic disease conditions and complicated prescription medicine regimens.

A woman at the front of the room asked, "Is there someone I could talk to after the workshop, about some of the medications I'm taking?" She had arrived about twenty minutes early and had diligently filled out all the surveys and release forms, and even started on a neighborhood mapping activity that participants would complete in small groups later in the workshop. I felt the room turn toward me, waiting for a response.

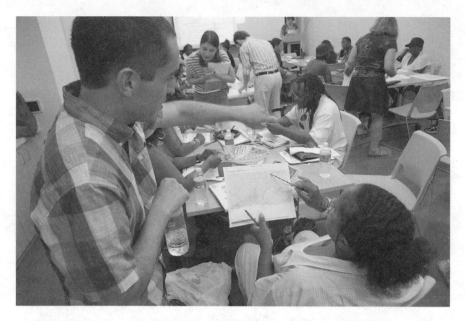

Russ Zerbo works with a participant engaged in a neighborhood mapping activity during the "Staying Cool in a Changing Climate" workshop held at the South Philadelphia branch of the Free Library, July 2017. Photograph by Richard Johnson.

"You know, we don't have any medical providers here today. There aren't any doctors or nurses on our project team. But I'm going to make a note of it for our next workshop. It would be good to have someone here who could answer some basic questions about medication and environment." I looked to the other facilitators and nodded to signal that we should discuss this after the workshop. Since this was the fourth year we had offered the Climate, Health, and Home series of workshops, the facilitators were able to anticipate most of the questions that participants might have about local environmental health issues. Sometimes, though, they still stumped us. Perhaps next time we could invite someone from Physicians for Social Responsibility or Drexel's School of Medicine, I thought, if PDPH or the National Nurse-Led Care Consortium (NNCC) had no one available on staff who could join us.

The "Staying Cool in a Changing Climate" workshop was designed and hosted by a team of people from six Philadelphia-based organizations involved with the larger Climate, Health, and Home project: the Clean Air Council, Drexel University, the Energy Coordinating Agency, Liberty Lutheran, NNCC, and PDPH. Each organization contributed specialized content to the climate- and health-focused project. The Clean Air Council provided an environmental justice focus and brought several years of experience in giving presentations on climate change in Philadelphia. The Energy Coordinating Agency discussed energy efficiency in the home and its relationship to climate change and weather. This paired well with information from NNCC's Healthy Homes Program, which focused on how indoor environments affect family health. Liberty Lutheran, an elder-care organization serving southeastern Pennsylvania, helped participants strategize preparation for extreme weather events at home and surveyed the governmental and nongovernmental resources available to senior citizens. PDPH provided a detailed description of the health impacts of heat health emergencies and outlined the city's responses to these events.

My role as a social scientist was to provide an overview of the project, moderate the discussion, and facilitate activities. Within the context of the larger project, I collected data on participants' existing knowledge of climate change and health impacts, energy efficiency practices, and city services and also produced publicly accessible curricula that could be shared with other organizations. Workshop participants received a "health kit" from PDPH as well as a folder with information from each presentation, resource flyers, and a twenty-five-dollar gift card as an expression of the team's gratitude for participating in the project. Over a span of four years, the team facilitated nine workshops in eight Philadelphia locations. More than two hundred people had participated in the Climate, Health, and Home workshop series at the time of this writing.

The broader Climate, Health, and Home project was funded by the Climate and Urban Systems Partnership (CUSP), a multicity network funded by a five-year National Science Foundation grant and a driving force behind many Philadelphia-based climate change initiatives. As the lead CUSP organization in Philadelphia, the Franklin Institute, a long-standing science museum, has been tasked with building a robust network of climate change educators through organizational partnerships across the city.[13] With nearly a hundred member organizations, CUSP experiments with innovative, community-based strategies that educate citizens about climate change and its local impacts. More than fifty climate education programs involving collaborative teams of experimenters have been hosted in Philadelphia alone. CUSP's mini-grant program, which provided four years of funding for the Climate, Health, and Home project, is just one of the many ways in which the Franklin Institute builds the CUSP network. Other tactics include monthly webinars, quarterly networking events, support for collaborative tabling at festivals, and distribution of climate kits that member organizations can use for demonstrations in interactive workshops.

All of these activities support initiatives that address climate change in ways specific to Philadelphia and emphasize building collective responses to climate change in local communities.

Each year, the Climate, Health, and Home team grew as we collaborated with different organizations to refine workshop content, create new activities, and address specialized themes. As the project name suggests, the core curriculum addressed the impact of climate change on both public and home environments in Philadelphia, especially how people with asthma may be affected by new environmental conditions. When we launched the project in 2014, our goal was to adapt information and resources from NNCC's Healthy Homes Program for the context of climate change in Philadelphia. "Healthy homes" initiatives are public health interventions that have slowly been institutionalized across the United States over the past twenty-five years, thanks to federal legislation that provides program funding through the U.S. Department of Housing and Urban Development. Often found in urban areas, healthy homes programs are anchored by community health workers who visit low-income families in their homes. These health workers provide in-home assessments and education to families with children diagnosed with asthma and other environmental illnesses, such as exposure to lead. Healthy homes programs have become a pillar of public health campaigns addressing the urban asthma epidemic.

The third presenter at our "Staying Cool in a Changing Climate" workshop, Deepa Mankikar from NNCC, asked participants if they had thought about how climate change would affect their home environments. One person yelled out, "Mold," a cry that echoed through the room as other people chimed in. "Mold is everywhere and it can kill you," a man boomed from the back of the room. "I've had asthma my whole life and I feel like I've noticed mold more in recent years. It's everywhere." A woman said that she had to move because the mold in her apartment was so bad: "It was all over the closet and the bathroom. I was wondering why I wasn't feeling good. I couldn't see it, but I could smell it and feel it in the air. Then they moved me to a new apartment at Eighth and Locust and now I can breathe better. It feels so good, you can notice the difference." Unfortunately, this woman's experience is an exception; most Philadelphians in senior housing face long waits if they need to move.

The workshop participants had learned about the event through flyers and e-mails that went out to community centers and municipal agencies, as well as by word of mouth. All of the project partners additionally promoted the workshop through their own organizational channels. Russ Zerbo, for instance, distributed flyers at public libraries and monthly community meetings to get the word out in the neighborhoods where our workshops would be held. This broad, community-based approach to event promotion meant that we never quite knew who to expect at our workshops. Participants had to provide their zip codes when they registered in advance, so we knew that we could expect participants from far and wide. Almost all workshop participants were African American seniors, with more women attending than men, but the demographics varied slightly across workshop locations.

Participants' living situations varied, too. Some participants owned their own homes (and had for decades), while others rented or lived in senior housing. A handful of participants were experiencing homelessness at the time of the workshop. As facilitators, we needed to be able to talk about climate change and health across different housing situations. People experiencing homelessness, for example, needed to hear about the city's Code Red services, which are activated before a heat health emergency and are designed to address the specific vulnerabilities associated with homelessness. Similarly, renters had needs and experiences that were different from those of homeowners. At each workshop we heard how vulnerable renters are to the whims and absences of landlords. Renters had few options for addressing mold or increasing ventilation. Many of the homeowners who attended our workshops were retired, and those who were still working had low incomes, which meant that they lacked the resources to make any major modifications to their homes, even though they had the authority to do so. The workshops had to strike a balance between suggesting tactics that participants could implement on their own and pointing people to governmental and nongovernmental resources.

Because the workshops were the products of collaboration among organizations from many different sectors, involving people whose expertise and resources addressed climate change from a variety of angles, the facilitators could offer wide-ranging information on home environments, public spaces, and city resources. Before this project began, most of this information was situated in specific domains, with little overlap among them. The structure provided by the CUSP program, combined with other local and federal climate change initiatives, provided opportunities for the organizations involved to partner and piece together resources in new ways. Indeed, one of the many goals of the Climate, Health, and Home project was to draw these resources and information sets together into a kind of tool kit for organizations and citizens.[14]

As a collaborative endeavor involving different kinds of expertise and services, the work conducted by the Climate, Health, and Home team exemplifies the production of a carescape that can help address asthma through public health arenas. Feminist geographer Sophie Bowlby uses the term *caringscapes* to describe how care is enacted in different tempo-ralities and terrains over the life course. It reflects how the dynamics of an individual's situation and needs change over time and place. A person may experience changes in income, for example, and in health status. Living situations and social relations change as well, sometimes from year to year and certainly over decades. Bowlby also develops the concept of care-scapes, which encompass the broader "resource and service context" that shapes people's ability to care. Caringscapes and carescapes are entangled with various sociocultural scales, including local and national economies, new public policies, and emerging technologies. The dynamic interplay be-tween these scales creates "spaces of care that might be regarded as fixed over the short term [but] are subject to change as a result of processes operating over time-space."[15] The connection between the caringscapes, or how an individual's life position changes over time, and the political or institutional carescapes that shape care practices allows us to make sense of "nested dependencies" of care.[16] This nested structure is particularly salient for thinking about elder care, for example, or about the public health programs that address the asthma epidemic in cities. It can also be a powerful tool for anticipating the effects of climate change in relation to existing social, political, and health vulnerabilities.

The relationship between caringscapes and carescapes is one way to think about how the Climate, Health, and Home project team structured workshop content, bridging the realms of public and private resources in the face of local climate change impacts. A key thrust of the workshops was to help participants think about the relationship between their homes and existing caringscapes and the Philadelphia carescape emerging to address asthma anew, in the context of climate change, which included a range of governmental and nongovernmental resources. For me, Bowlby's framework became a way to think about the larger public health care-scape emerging in Philadelphia as well as the national health impacts of climate change.

The Changing Atmosphere of Asthma Triggers

Lily Davis, a seventy-two-year-old African American woman, had lived in her West Philadelphia neighborhood for more than seven decades. She attended the "Staying Cool in a Changing Climate" workshop in June 2017, the first time we offered it at the West Philadelphia Senior Commu-nity Center. Lily had been a member of the center for a number of years, ever since she retired from her position at one of Philadelphia's munici-pal agencies. She was one of more than thirty people who, at the end of the workshop, signed up to participate in our postworkshop interviews. These interviews were a new addition to the Climate, Health, and Home project. They were different in a number of ways from the interviews I had conducted years earlier for my research on asthma care. For one thing, Russ Zerbo and I conducted them collaboratively. Instead of asking questions specifically related to asthma, we used an oral history format and asked participants about their understanding of and concerns with climate change, as well as their experience of environment, housing, and city services.

As in the workshops, asthma came up in the interviews even when we did not ask about it. When I asked Lily if there were any environmental changes that stood out to her, in her experience living in Philadelphia for the past seventy years, her response came from an emplaced perspective on the relationship between climate change and urban development:

> The weather I'm really not understanding, because you used to be able to—I'm going to use the word "predict" what was coming on with the weather. Like, right now, I have a broken bone, so I'm a walking thermometer right now. And it hurts, hurts, hurts. But you had coal stoves, and we heated the homes by coal. And then it changed to oil, and you would see a lot of smog and what have you. But I think because we had a lot of grass and trees and other plants that would clean the air for us, it wasn't as bad. It wasn't as bad. Now, the grounds are being taken for "development," quote unquote. And it's hurting everybody. I developed asthma at a late age, and I thought they made a mistake. So, they sent me to two other doctors, and they said, no, you have asthma. I said, that's impossible, I'm thirty-three years old, why would I have asthma now? But I was in an area where there were a lot of cars, you know, I was on my own. Cars going by, my windows were always open, so anytime anything went by with that fuel, you could smell it. That's when I would start the hacking. And if our season is changing between winter and summer, it would be really, really bad. And once it became cold, fine. Or once it became hot and stayed, fine. But that in-between stage, the pollen was high and as I said, the vehicles were there, blowing out smoke.

Weather was often one of the first things that came up when we asked people about environmental change. They also frequently mentioned gentrification and development. Neither of these latter two topics was explicitly on the agenda either, but we found that West Philadelphia seniors, most of whom had lived their entire lives in what was now a gentrified and gentrifying district, had a great deal to say about the interrelated changes in the built and natural environment. For Lily, weather, air quality, traffic, and development were all layered together in her emplaced experience. She could feel the weather and the seasons change in her body—in the broken bone in her arm and also in her breathing—but she linked this to "development" and the car pollution that came into her home.[17] Development had changed the environment, and it was hurting everybody.

John, an African American man in his seventies who had lived in Philadelphia off and on his entire adult life, attended our July workshop at the South Philadelphia branch of the Free Library. John worked with people experiencing homelessness, and he had an in-depth knowledge of the issues that came up on the streets and in public places, where the people he worked with were continually exposed to the outdoor environment. John had good working knowledge of climate change before he participated in the workshop. During our postworkshop interview, when we talked about new things he learned from the session, he said that he appreciated learning about, as he put it, "the state of Philadelphia." He noted that the local information shared in the presentations—on air quality data and city services—had not received as much publicity as the information about global climate change:

> But yeah, so I learned where to go. But also, about the concerns of
> other people. I work with a lot of people who have asthma. The pollen
> in this area. That's one thing I've noticed as I get older, allergies are
> starting to get bad and pollen in particular. I've learned, kind of keeping
> up with the state of Philadelphia, about the pollen index and that kind
> of thing. The places to go, and other kind of things.

I asked John how the environment had changed over time, in the decades that he had lived in Philadelphia.

> Just hanging about the Schuylkill [River], I've noticed just the pollen
> index. I mean, besides the construction, just how hard it is to breathe
> in Center City. It's hard to breathe in Center City. Just walking around,
> I think that—I guess with all of the construction, but also just the
> pollen index is so bad there and whatever. And like I said, I just
> attribute it to a lot of construction and a lot of dust, which is all over
> the place. But I think it's also the level of heat that makes it harder to
> breathe. And working with the homeless population for the nonprofit,
> how the quality of just the breathing stuff, it's really a danger to them.
> So, I work with that population and seeing the effects of it, and
> heatstroke, and people with diabetes, and in particular I spent some
> time in the dialysis center, I noticed the heat and how it affects them.
> So yeah, those kinds of things come out. The craziness of storms. It's

unpredictable. You know, seeing an increase of mosquitoes lately. I think Philadelphia is not a healthy city and hopefully they get back into that state [of health]. It's gotten worse in recent years. I used to walk around a lot and I need to get back to biking, I haven't done that, but I love walking around the city. I just noticed now, it's hard to breathe. I have to stop and avoid some places, and it just seems like it's harder. If I don't have water there, it will get constricted in my throat. It's getting worse, it seems to me.

Although John did not have asthma, he still had a hard time breathing in Philadelphia's busiest district, Center City, which is home to government offices, international corporations, the convention center, entertainment venues, and the shops and restaurants that typically accompany a business district. An organization that tracks the amount and types of construction taking place in Center City found that more than twenty-nine high-rise projects were under way in 2017 alone. This number does not include smaller-scale and older construction projects that have become part of the district's landscape. The uptick in construction has had profound impacts on Philadelphians who are experiencing homelessness.[18] Like Lily, John talked about air quality, but he saw it as a combination of things, including pollen, construction dust, and heat. He thought construction specifically contributed to worsening air quality and mentioned the development happening throughout Center City several times.

In these interviews, we specifically asked about environmental changes over time, invoking people's experience of timescapes, such as how their neighborhoods and atmospheres had changed over the course of their lives. Their emplaced responses drew on embodied experiences of breathing in Philadelphia's spaces that included riding public transportation, walking on specific streets, living in neighborhoods next to industry, and even just sitting at home with windows open to the unbreathable world. While the breathers in my earlier round of interviews frequently mentioned specific asthma triggers, Philadelphia seniors highlighted disordered breathing in atmospheres and environmental conditions that exceeded any one object or trigger.[19] Collectively, these responses clearly articulated how the asthma epidemic is produced by material legacies, infrastructures, and entanglements that are rendered invisible by the language of "triggers" in biomedicalized asthma care arenas. For example, the language of triggers renders invisible the structural inequalities and contexts of environmental racism, which have been linked to higher asthma prevalence rates and worse treatment outcomes in many cities.[20] As a single object or entity, a trigger invokes a narrow focus, one that can easily be made the responsibility of an individual, who must guard against exposure by keeping dust and pollen out of the home, for example, or by avoiding certain activities or places.

Climate change, however, is forcing a shift in how public health workers talk about asthma. In publications that discuss the potential impacts of climate change on the U.S. asthma epidemic, environmental health scientists have begun to expand from the language of triggers to a broader language of environments and atmospheres. Rather than presenting one-to-one relationships in which specific objects (cold air, dander, dust, smoke, pollen) trigger asthma symptoms, scientists are increasingly positioning disordered breathing contextually, referencing the complexity of ecosystems, atmospheres, and temporal changes.

This new, greater embrace of complexity is evidenced by the U.S. Global Change Research Program's April 2016 report *The Impacts of Climate Change on Human Health in the United States: A Scientific Assessment*.[21] This sweeping, evidence-based document is the first to map out the health impacts of climate change in depth and in detail. More than one hundred experts from federal agencies contributed to the report, which underwent extensive scientific and public review before its release. The report situates classic asthma triggers such as mold, pollen, and ozone in changing atmospheric conditions that involve many elements and relationships, including rising levels of carbon dioxide, increased precipitation, and urban heat islands. The document's more than three hundred pages cover a wide range of topics, including vector-borne diseases, food safety, extreme events, and mental health. In the chapter on air quality, where most of the information on asthma is located, the authors underscore how the complexity of a changing atmosphere makes asthma more difficult to manage. Our experience of the atmosphere has always been multidimensional, of course: temperature, wind speed, pollution density, time of day and year, humidity, and barometric pressure all factor into the quality of air. What makes climate change significant for people with breathing disorders is that familiar atmospheric patterns and conditions may be joined by new and unpredictable ones. For some asthma sufferers, this will make attunement a less reliable mode of care.

The allergenicity of plants, for example, is increasing with rising levels of carbon dioxide, warmer temperatures, and increased precipitation (in some regions of the United States). Allergenicity is a measure of how much a particular allergen, such as pollen, affects people. Ragweed allergenicity, for example, may increase from year to year, making people more sensitive when next exposed. The greater the allergenicity of pollen, the greater the severity and prevalence of pollen allergy across the population. This is different from the concentration of pollen in a specific location (the pollen count) or the length of the pollen season, both of which also affect the severity and prevalence of allergy in populations. These latter two dimensions—pollen count and pollen season—are what people most often refer to when discussing the relationship between pollen and climate change. Indeed, many weather apps and websites offer "allergy forecasts" that show daily pollen counts by zip code. John, for example, checked the pollen levels in his local area each day: "Usually when I check the weather, I look at the pollen, because it's there on AccuWeather when I check it. I kind of get the idea of what I'm venturing out to, just when I walk around the city. Like, here, I walked down here. So, I keep an eye out, but I usually check it every day." Information on pollen allergenicity, in contrast, is less accessible to laypersons.

The report by the U.S. Global Change Research Program (USGCRP) emphasizes that public health organizations need to consider and prepare for the changing ways in which allergens are becoming emplaced and related to other environmental, infrastructural, and socioeconomic factors. In the chapter titled "Air Quality Impacts," the authors point to numerous environmental and atmospheric dynamics that can play into the exacerbation of allergic diseases, including asthma:

> Climate change related alterations in local weather patterns, including changes in minimum and maximum temperatures and rainfall, affect the burden of allergic diseases. The role of weather on the initiation or exacerbation of allergic symptoms in sensitive persons is not well understood. So-called "thunderstorm asthma" results as allergenic particles are dispersed through osmotic rupture, a phenomenon where cell membranes burst. Pollen grains may, after contact with rain, release part of their cellular contents, including allergen-laced fine particles. Increases in the intensity and frequency of heavy rainfall and storminess over the coming decades is likely to be associated with spikes in aeroallergen concentrations and the potential for related increases in the number and severity of allergic illnesses.
>
> Potential non-linear interactions between aeroallergens and ambient air pollutants (including ozone, nitrogen dioxide, sulfur dioxide, and fine particulate matter) may increase health risks for people who are simultaneously exposed. In particular, pre-exposure to air pollution (especially ozone or fine particulate matter) may magnify the effects of aeroallergens, as prior damage to airways may increase the permeability of mucous membranes to the penetration of allergens, although existing evidence suggests greater sensitivity but not necessarily a direct link with ozone exposure. A recent report noted remaining uncertainties across the epidemiologic, controlled human exposure, and toxicology studies on this emerging topic.[22]

Because weather conditions can interact with pollen behavior in unpre-dictable ways, it may be risky for breathers to rely on existing attunement and breath control practices alone. The report's authors cite thunderstorm asthma as an example of a new kind of atmospheric event, the conditions and severity of which are different from what people have experienced in the past.[23] But the changes are not limited to weather. "Non-linear inter-actions" between pollution and pollen will also impact breathers. The authors note that the temporal sequence of atmospheric exposures and their effects on the body may be important for sensitized breathers, but in ways as yet unknown. Legacy airway damage and sensitization also matter for how breathers may be triggered by such acute events as thunderstorm asthma, intensified pollen seasons, and heat health emergencies that come with high concentrations of ground-level ozone. The big takeaway from the USGCRP report—beyond its extensive description of environmental health changes backed by rigorous research—is its discursive framing of asthma as a public health problem that goes beyond a list of triggers. Emplacing asthma in climate change allows public health agencies to take actions that address the epidemic beyond individual control strategies.

While the USGCRP report provides extensive documentation of the problem and specifies where more research is needed, it does not make programmatic recommendations, nor does it gesture toward solutions. Instead, it offers a diligent, evidence-based survey of the complexity of cli-mate change from a public health perspective, a great feat in itself. Other federal agencies, however, have stepped in to create programs and work toward solutions. The Centers for Disease Control and Prevention, for example, established its Climate and Health Program in 2009. The pro-gram's threefold aim is to identify populations vulnerable to climate change, to prevent and adapt to the health impacts of climate change, and to build systems to detect and respond to potential health threats related to climate change.[24] At the time of this writing, one of the CDC's core programs is its Climate-Ready States and Cities Initiative, which provides resources and a policy structure to help city and state health departments address climate vulnerabilities. This includes using climate science to predict local impacts on health and creating flexible climate programs based on existing and emerging data. The CDC's programs focus on modeling and monitor-ing population health in relation to environmental conditions—a necessary first step in planning for climate change. The programs emphasize popula-tion health surveillance systems cued into such environmental dynamics as air quality. The CDC also encourages municipalities and state health departments to create climate and health adaptation plans, a process that ideally involves a multitude of stakeholders. Nonprofit foundations, too, have begun to fund urban climate and health initiatives globally and in the United States. In my work at the intersection of climate change and health, I have seen the CDC's resources taken up in a variety of ways by local and state organizations, including the Philadelphia Department of Public Health. Indeed, PDPH has taken the lead in cultivating an asthma carescape that can address the conditions of climate change.

In 2015, PDPH received a grant from the Public Health Institute for its Asthma Readiness and Resilience Project, the goal of which is to develop a climate change–focused curriculum for asthma sufferers in Philadelphia.[25] As part of the project, PDPH plans to develop a public notification system to alert asthma sufferers when weather and air quality conditions are likely to produce symptoms. In addition to this grant project, PDPH convened a climate and health advisory group, with representatives from more than forty Philadelphia organizations, to advise PDPH on developing a citywide climate and health adaptation plan. PDPH's climate and health project manager, Jessica Caum, also convened two special working

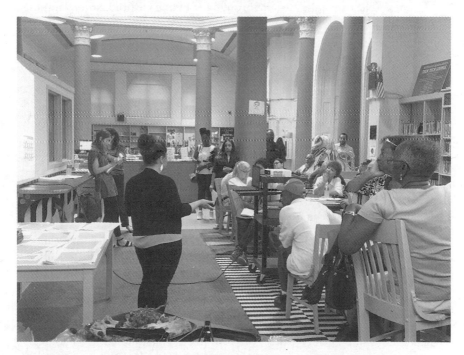

Maria Ramirez of the Philadelphia Department of Public Health describes heat health emergencies during the "Staying Cool in a Changing Climate" workshop held at the McPherson Library in Philadelphia, August 2017. Photograph by Deepa Mankikar.

groups to address population health vulnerabilities that needed more concerted attention and immediate action: one on climate and asthma, and a
second on extreme heat. One outcome of the climate and health advisory
group's work was PDPH's updated heat health emergency plan, which
was presented at the community workshops described above.

Carescapes is a term useful for describing how organizations, resources,
and policies are knit together in relations of care. In this case, the emergent carescape produced explanations of climate science that used local
environmental data, established locally relevant public services, brought
expert organizations from different sectors to the same table, and retooled
existing programs to respond to new needs. The PDPH climate and asthma
working group, for example, included not only partners from Philadelphia's existing asthma carescape—health care workers from several hospitals, representatives from healthy homes programs, and staff members
from the school district—but also members of environmental justice organizations, representatives of other municipal agencies, and university researchers. The carescape created through the Public Health Institute grant,
CUSP, and the city's climate and health advisory groups helped get information out to communities in new ways as well. PDPH has used CUSP and
the existing asthma care network in Philadelphia to get both professional
and public feedback on curriculum, share data, and conduct outreach to
distribute new information and materials. Carescapes are patchworks of
existing and emerging elements. In the case of Philadelphia's climate carescape, the existing asthma epidemic—connected as it is to deep poverty,
poor housing conditions, and inadequate school infrastructure (a topic to
which I will return later in this chapter)—provided a robust existing care
network to work with.

Making Healthy Homes from the Outside In

Fourteen women, two babies, and one man sat around tables in a semi-
circle facing a wall-sized screen. The presentation slide showed air pollution making its way into a home. The caption underneath the picture read,
"Protection from outdoor air reduces ventilation in the home." It was a
mixed message: if you leave your windows open, air pollution will come
inside; if you keep your windows closed, you reduce indoor ventilation and
make indoor air quality worse. We repeatedly encountered such double
binds as we tried to adapt content designed for healthy homes programs,
which focus on indoor environments, to the dynamics of climate change.

The "Be Air Aware" workshop was the very first event hosted by the
Climate, Health, and Home team. Held in September 2014, the workshop

was attended primarily by African American women who lived in the neighborhoods of West Philadelphia, Kensington, and North Philadelphia. This first workshop, held in the River Wards city planning district, had been offered to new mothers and their families through one of NNCC's local programs. Like most of the subsequent Climate, Health, and Home workshops, it ran for two hours and included group discussion, short presentations, and hands-on activities. Since the project began before the USGCRP report was published, this first workshop tracked back and forth between known triggers such as mold, ozone, and domestic chemicals and climate change effects such as urban heat islands, increases in precipitation, and extreme weather events.

The breathability of indoor environments is complicated by extreme heat events, in that businesses and residents have to either open their windows or turn on air-conditioning to stay cool. At the workshop, Saleem Chapman from the Clean Air Council described how rising summer temperatures turn Philadelphia into an urban heat island. Concrete landscapes and heat-absorbing rooftops capture and contain heat, especially in dense neighborhoods that lack parks and trees. Air conditioners, Saleem told the group, contribute to the heat island by kicking hot air out into the atmosphere and demanding more energy across the power grid. But, he continued, the problems with heat islands go beyond just temperature. An urban heat island produces more ground-level ozone as well. This is a huge concern for breathers, since "current levels of ground-level ozone have been estimated to be responsible for tens of thousands of hospital and emergency room visits, millions of cases of acute respiratory symptoms and school absences, and thousands of premature deaths each year in the United States," according to the USGCRP report.[26] The effect happens indoors as well as outside, as air pollution seeps in through open windows and doors. People who use fans to keep their homes cool during the summer are especially vulnerable. This was the case for many of our workshop participants.

Climate change research, including work summarized in the USGCRP report, gives a rich perspective on the connection between outdoor and indoor climates. Most people spend a majority of their time—up to 90 percent, according to multiple studies cited in the report—indoors.[27] This makes the condition of built environments a core determinant of health, and, indeed, indoor environments have been a significant focus of asthma research.[28] Increased concentrations of outdoor air pollution, such as ground-level ozone, dust, pollen, and particulate matter, may result in more of this material finding its way inside homes. But when people keep their houses closed up, they decrease ventilation, allowing indoor pollutants such as mold, carbon monoxide, volatile organic compounds, and formaldehyde to build up. Windows, in this context, operate as a double bind that signals deeper structural issues. With its aging housing stock, Philadelphia faces a particular threat from mold. In some areas of the city, including portions of the River Wards, flooding has been a long-standing issue; more intense precipitation events mean more water damage for many people. The USGCRP report notes that "dampness and mold in U.S. homes are linked to approximately 4.6 million cases of worsened asthma and between 8% and 20% of several common respiratory infections, such as acute bronchitis."[29]

Our mixed-message slide put the trade-offs of indoor and outdoor pollution side by side. Although some workshop participants had air-conditioning, many opened their windows and used fans to keep their homes cool. Such ventilation during heat waves could bring ozone, particulate matter, and pollen into indoor breathing spaces. Stagnant air, on the other hand, could lead to a buildup of asthma triggers like dust, dander, domestic chemicals, and conditions that breed mold. And how many people want to keep their homes sealed up during summer anyway? At a glance, it might have seemed as if we were pointing to danger in both directions: damned if you do, damned if you don't. But as participants described the constraints of their home environments, I felt like our slide opened the door to a discussion of a much larger set of structural issues.

One woman explained that her bathroom was a former closet that had been converted years earlier when the building's owner had divided the house into multiple units. With no exhaust fan or windows (an unenforced code violation), the bathroom had accumulated black mold on the ceiling and walls. Another woman said that outdoor ventilation was not an option for her in every room. The windows in her bedroom and kitchen were sealed shut; try as she might, she could not get them open. One of the older women attending the workshop, who had come with her daughter, chimed in: "I have lived in apartments where my windows are sealed shut, too. Painted over. The problem is the landlords. They don't care. They won't do anything to fix it." We listened as the women related the different dilemmas they faced, and were frustrated by, in their home environments. In this first workshop, I was hearing such descriptions for the first time, but to our NNCC collaborators the stories the women told of the conditions in Philadelphia's low-income housing landscape were familiar, if unacceptable.

Shawana, a community health worker who anchored NNCC's Healthy Homes Program, responded to questions about the outdoor–indoor pollution slide, pointing participants to resources and suggesting things to try in the home. She described how to arrange fans to get a cross breeze and pointed participants to AirNow, an air quality forecasting service managed by the U.S. Environmental Protection Agency. Saleem then brought up the next slide, which showed the EPA's Air Quality Index as it appears on the AirNow website. He walked participants through the color-coded scale, explaining that the lower the segment, the higher the level of air pollution. When the air quality falls into the orange segment, for example, that means the pollution level is in the range of 101 to 150 on the AQI scale of 0 to 500; the EPA categorizes this level as unhealthy for sensitive groups such as children, the elderly, and people with respiratory diseases like asthma. Air quality that falls into the red segment on the scale is considered unhealthy for everyone. On days when pollution reaches this level, people should stay indoors if possible.[30] Shawana also encouraged participants to think about where they live, which also matters. If you live next to a highway, she explained, you should not have your windows open during heavy traffic periods, such as morning commute hours.

Shawana reminded participants that they should change the air filters in their air conditioners regularly and that they should be sure to periodically inspect areas susceptible to mold, such as bathrooms, the spaces under and around sinks, and basements, if they had access. She also provided contact information for a city office where participants could access legal counsel if they had problems with negligent or absentee landlords. Several of the participants lit up when Shawana mentioned this office, and one woman asked her to repeat the information as many in the room wrote it down in the notes section of their workshop packet. Clearly, at our next workshop we needed to include the office's contact details in the packet we gave to participants. As the Climate, Health, and Home team would learn over the years, one of the components of our workshops that was most valuable to participants was the information we provided on governmental and nongovernmental programs that might offer assistance with their homes. While some of the suggestions Shawana offered were intuitive, others were the result of things she had learned through years of working in NNCC's Philadelphia-based Healthy Homes Program.

Shawana's expertise as a community health worker focused on childhood asthma and lead poisoning and derived from her work in Philadelphia homes for almost ten years. Community health workers have been described as "frontline public health workers" who serve as liaisons to health and social services, provide health education and advocacy, and conduct outreach in communities.[31] Community health workers play a particularly important role in healthy homes programs, which originated as an extension of the lead hazard control programs established in the

1990s under Title X of the Housing and Community Development Act of 1992.[32] In 1999, Congress expanded these lead-focused programs to encompass a broader array of childhood environmental hazards, including mold, pests, dust mites, pesticides, asbestos, radon, and carbon monoxide, as well as general home safety issues. NNCC's state-funded Healthy Homes Program sends community health workers out to visit the homes of low-income families whose children have been diagnosed with asthma or have been found through testing to have blood lead levels that exceed safe amounts. During an asthma-related family home visit, the community health worker uses several standardized surveys to conduct an assessment of the environmental health conditions present and then recommends material alterations that the family can make to reduce children's exposures to asthma triggers. For instance, the health worker may suggest addressing areas that leak water and breed mold, patching places where pests can enter and find food, or even replacing items and surfaces that might capture and retain dust easily, such as curtains, rugs, and pillows. The idea is to educate the family about "environmental control" strategies that, when coupled with medication adherence, can increase asthma control.[33] After the initial visit, the community health worker makes one or more follow-up visits over three to six months (the number and timing of these visits can vary) to assess how well the family has implemented the recommendations and to help troubleshoot any problems.

The Climate, Health, and Home project translated materials from the NNCC Healthy Homes Program into a public presentation, with information sheets and care kits that participants could take home with them. During the workshop itself, participants learned how to make cleaning products at home using lemon juice, baking soda, and water. The workshop also included a home mapping activity that helped participants to identify areas in their homes with existing or potential air quality problems. Some participants used this activity to explore do-it-yourself ventilation strategies, while others used their maps to think through their home environments in terms of asthma triggers. At the end of the workshop, participants went home with "blackout" curtains to keep their homes cool, charcoal dehumidifiers for bathrooms, and the cleaning solution that they had concocted during the session.

In our 2014 workshops, the Climate, Health, and Home team's focus was threefold: to build cross-sectoral partnerships among the Clean Air Council, NNCC, and Drexel University; to create spaces where community members and project team members could engage in two-way learning about the local impacts of climate change in Philadelphia; and to adapt healthy homes program content, which is traditionally disseminated in

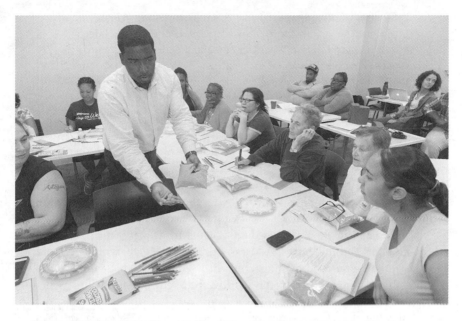

Saleem Chapman of the Clean Air Council explains the dangers of mold and humidity to participants in the "Be Air Aware" workshop presented by the Climate, Health, and Home project, September 2014. Photograph by Mark Garvin.

private homes, to a format for public dissemination. Some observers might criticize this approach as too limited, arguing, for example, that coaching persons living in poverty on how to use charcoal dehumidifiers distracts from the larger political struggles that might address some of the root causes of climate change. Indeed, during our 2015 workshop series, some participants pointed to the limitations of our approach—after all, teaching people to make their own household cleaning products will not force policy makers to do their jobs, nor will such tactics solve the problem of landlord negligence. Our broad goal in conducting the workshops, however, was of necessity more modest: to adjust the asthma carescape in Philadelphia so that it would provide vulnerable residents with the resources they needed to learn about and engage with climate change on terms that were meaningful in the context of their lives.[34]

We ended each workshop with a group discussion of the takeaways from the presentation and the activities. Everyone liked making the all-purpose cleaner, and most thought the mapping activity was useful. The interactive components were always among participants' favorite parts. One of the participants, Barbara, explained why these activities were effective:

> Before this workshop, when I hear "environment" I just shut down. Environment is too big for me. Environment is out there and I don't have any control over it. What can I do about pollution? How am I supposed to save the whales? Or whatever. Environment is expensive too! Taking care of the environment is expensive! But I like how this workshop makes it about things I can do in my home. Simple things that I can afford.

"Yeah, it's like you have to go big or go home," Sherrilynn, another workshop participant, agreed. The participants felt that addressing environmental issues in the ways conveyed by mainstream advertisements and conservation campaigns was beyond what they could contribute, whether financially or in their daily lives. Being "environmentally friendly" was expensive, and it often seemed disconnected from the participants' own communities and daily lives. Addressing climate change, with its popular focus on the fate of drowning polar bears, fell into this category too. Another woman added that the workshop taught her about things that mattered to her, like making sure the house was healthy for her kids.

"And hopefully today you got a better understanding of the relationship between the big environment and the home environment," Saleem replied. "That what's happening with climate change. What's going on with the big environment will impact your home environment and your neighborhood." Helping people make connections between climate change and what was going on in their own lives and communities was at the core of the goals of CUSP, the larger project that funded our workshops.

Unbreathable

Laporshia Massey died of an asthma attack on September 26, 2013. She was twelve years old and a lifelong Philadelphia resident. She attended W. C. Bryant Promise Academy, a K–8 school run by the School District of Philadelphia. Early in the afternoon on the day she died, Laporshia reported breathing difficulty to her teacher, but she never used a rescue inhaler at school that day. Media reports of her death did not indicate whether one was available or not. Their main focus, rather, was on the absence of the school nurse, who worked at W. C. Bryant only two days a week and was not on duty on September 26.[35] After school, a staff member drove Laporshia home because she was continuing to have an asthma attack. At this point, hours had gone by since Laporshia had first told her teacher she could not breathe. Later that afternoon, Laporshia's father set out to drive her to the emergency room at Children's Hospital of

Philadelphia, but she stopped breathing on the way there. Her panicked father flagged down paramedics roadside, but Laporshia was pronounced dead at the hospital.

Most news reports on Laporshia Massey's death focused on the problem of caregiving in schools. Philadelphia's underfunded school district has long struggled with staffing its schools with any more than "essential" staff, and the fall 2013 school year started after a particularly brutal round of budget cuts. All summer long, child advocates had warned that something like this would happen. One report describing the lawsuit that followed Laporshia's death stated that students at W. C. Bryant were not allowed to use inhalers without a nurse present, a rule at odds with school district and state policy.[36] Unable to administer her inhaler, Laporshia's teacher told the girl to "stay calm" in the face of her attack. Some news reports asked why the child was not taken to the emergency room immediately. Why did no one call 911? The school defended itself by saying that it tried to contact Laporshia's father twice, but could not reach him—a not uncommon situation for working parents. By all accounts, at least three to four adult caregivers (teacher, other school staff, and father) misjudged the severity of Laporshia's attack. Considering the number of children with asthma in Philadelphia, disordered breathing is presumably a common part of school culture at W. C. Bryant.

Tyra Bryant-Stephens, a doctor and medical director of the Children's Hospital of Philadelphia's Community Asthma Prevention Program, established in 1997, has conducted community-based studies on asthma prevalence and care in West and North Philadelphia. Her research shows that the screening protocols used in local, regional, and state assessments often miss asthma sufferers in high-risk areas, resulting in underestimates of the prevalence of the disease.[37] The standard school screening programs that Bryant-Stephens and her colleagues have studied, for example, put childhood asthma prevalence at 25.7 percent in the neighborhoods assessed, compared to a county-wide rate of 22 percent. But door-to-door screening conducted by the researchers found childhood asthma rates to be higher than reported based on the standard screening methods—in the cases of neighborhoods with the highest poverty rates, much higher. In the two Philadelphia zip codes with the highest percentages of children living in poverty, the researchers found asthma prevalence rates as high as 47.3 percent and 40.2 percent.[38] With prevalence rates so high, many cases of disordered breathing are most likely not being cared for and treated.

Part of the argument that Bryant-Stephens and her colleagues make is that most asthma research overlooks the most vulnerable breathers. There are a number of reasons for this. Medical researchers have difficulty recruiting and retaining vulnerable subjects, and they are reluctant to enroll study participants who experience complicating factors—such as comorbid medical conditions, deep poverty, and complex environmental stressors—that might confound the results. Even clinical researchers who work with vulnerable populations may underestimate the extent to which their patients experience disordered breathing, Bryant-Stephens and her colleagues argue. In a 2016 article, they document extensive environmental exposures and socioeconomic stressors in Philadelphia homes that other researchers have missed when they have failed to include analysis of home environments. In this particular study, community health workers made multiple in-home visits over a six-month period to assist with asthma care. In reporting on the study, Bryant-Stephens and her colleagues note that "even experienced asthma investigators have been dismayed by the depth of illness and poverty encountered during home visits."[39]

In Philadelphia, hazardous indoor environments are not limited to homes—they are also present in schools. Since Laporshia Massey's death in 2013, the Philadelphia Federation of Teachers and numerous other advocates have drawn attention to the deleterious conditions inside the city's schools. In a preliminary study conducted by the National Institute for Occupational Safety and Health, 60 percent of the thirty-six schools evaluated had dampness, mold, and water damage in more than one-third of the rooms. Additional rooms had mold or mold odor. At W. C. Bryant, the study found "water-related deterioration in 95.2 percent of the school's rooms."[40] Although reports indicate that the School District of Philadelphia halted the study before NIOSH could complete its assessment (the above numbers reflect visual assessment only), researchers were able to publish findings on a related study that investigated asthma rates among Philadelphia schoolteachers. Of the 1,136 teachers surveyed, nearly 10 percent reported that they were diagnosed with asthma after starting work in the school district.[41] More recent investigative news coverage has documented extensive mold, water damage, pest infestations, and peeling paint (which may contain lead) in Philadelphia schools.[42] As recently as August 2017, Muñoz-Marin Elementary School in North Philadelphia was hustling to eradicate an extensive mold outbreak that covered thousands of square feet of school surfaces, "even the mail slots in the main office." Another school, Roberto Clemente Middle School, also in North Philadelphia, had a mold outbreak as well. The district was paying more than $300,000 to get Muñoz-Marin ready for opening day, September 5.[43] Issues such as these have led to the formation of the Philly Healthy Schools Initiative, a coalition of seventeen organizations whose goal is to hold the school district accountable for the schools' environmental problems.

The city of Philadelphia has significant infrastructural issues to address, including issues related to deep poverty, structural racism, and antagonistic political relations with the state government that are having negative impacts on the existing Philadelphia carescape, not the least of which is the public school system. I end this chapter with Laporshia Massey's death, the dangerous conditions in Philadelphia schools, and the work of Tyra Bryant-Stephens and her colleagues to emphasize that efforts to address the impacts of climate change on asthma and its care need to start with the already existing conditions that have produced the epidemic in the first place. While the public health literature on asthma often lists triggers in linear form—a mode of representation I have mirrored throughout this book—recent governmental and scientific reports on the health impacts of climate change present a more complex, dynamic terrain for human–environment relations. As one potent example of this discursive shift, the USGCRP report draws on and knits together the findings of decades of public health research on asthma, which point to environmental degradation and poverty as the root causes of the U.S. epidemic.

As an environmental health problem, asthma provides a powerful example of how timescales, and slow violence in particular, make for unbreathable worlds. Rob Nixon, an interdisciplinary humanities scholar, defines slow violence as

> a violence that occurs gradually and out of sight, a violence of delayed destruction that is dispersed across time and space, an attritional violence that is typically not viewed as violence at all. Violence is customarily conceived as an event or action that is immediate in time, explosive and spectacular in space, and as erupting into instant sensational visibility. We need, I believe, to engage a different kind of violence, a violence that is neither spectacular nor instantaneous, but rather incremental and accretive, its calamitous repercussions playing out across a range of temporal scales. In so doing, we also need to engage the representational, narrative, and strategic challenges posed by the relative invisibility of slow violence.[44]

The image on the cover of Nixon's book *Slow Violence and the Environmentalism of the Poor* is one of smokestacks foregrounding a metropolitan skyline; when I first saw it, I thought it was a photograph of Philadelphia, taken from the River Wards. As it turned out, I was wrong, but even though the city depicted is not Philadelphia, the image reminds me of the layers of industry, aging working-class neighborhoods, and recent redevelopment projects (i.e., the construction that John and Lily mentioned) that have added to Philadelphia's asthmatic atmosphere. In his list of examples of environmental catastrophes and long dyings, Nixon names climate change first. I want to add the global asthma epidemic to Nixon's list, especially given the "representational, narrative, and strategic challenges" that it poses. Some of these challenges include asthma's multiple variants and its episodic tendencies; its relationship to environmental conditions, which include timescales ranging from a breath to the entire Anthropocene era; and the structural inequalities—in income, housing, and more—that Philadelphia policy makers, public health workers, and citizens face.

Addressing the slow violence of climate change and the global asthma epidemic requires new carescapes that are up to the task of dealing with an environmental health disease that is embedded within the condition of public infrastructure, including transportation corridors, zoning policies, housing, and even school buildings. It requires working across governmental, nonprofit, community, and educational sectors. It requires bringing public health and environmental justice campaigns together in new ways. After all, many of the people and places most vulnerable to climate change have been vulnerable since long before the turn toward preparing for new norms and extreme events.[45]

By the time I spoke with her, Lily Davis had lived with asthma for nearly forty years. When she has symptoms, she uses a rescue inhaler. She also keeps lots of plants in her apartment to improve the air quality of her indoor breathing space. I asked her if there was anything else she did, other tactics she used, to make her environment more breathable.

> I stay away from people who smoke, and I stay away from people who wear heavy colognes. If I was on SEPTA, I would really have a problem. Because you are getting on with all of these different scents, and you can't control it, there is absolutely nothing you can do about it, but sit there, and breathe through it. And pray. If I start coughing people will actually look at you, like, why are you on here with a cold? But it's not a cold. It's the air, you can't breathe. So, when I get like that I'll step off now. But it all depends on what I'm stepping into, because what's outside could be worse than what was inside. I just try to slow myself down and take a few deep breaths—in and out slowly, so that my lungs will have a chance to recuperate. I can't run the risk of having an asthma attack. It's safer for me, even weather-wise, to just go ahead and get off.

The Southeastern Pennsylvania Transportation Authority, or SEPTA, is Philadelphia's public transportation system; it includes buses, trolleys, various regional rail lines, and two subway routes. Lily described a scenario in which she has no control over her environmental exposure. Her symptoms are met with suspicious looks from other passengers, who do not understand why she cannot breathe. The other passengers do not realize that they all help to create a chemical cocktail that affects others, especially in a confined space where escape to a different breathing space may not be possible for several minutes. When this happens, Lily takes the next opportunity to exit, no matter where she is. The unknown risk of the outside environment—the air quality, the weather, the neighborhood—is better than the unbreathable space of the subway car or trolley.

Several modes of care come into view through Lily's experience of asthma on public transportation. The first is asthmatic attunement: Lily attunes to the atmosphere of the subway car, "getting on with all these scents," but she also takes in the looks from other passengers, an affective exchange in response to her cough. Attunement is anchored in an emplaced sense of relationships between the body and its surroundings. It is a way of being that draws on past experiences to situate and respond to present sensory information. Lily attunes to the atmosphere inside public transportation to determine whether she will be okay to travel to her destination.

Lily's account also highlights two ways that asthma sufferers most commonly attempt to exercise control. Lily has less control over her surroundings and exposures on SEPTA than she has at home, at work, or even in the social spaces that she frequents. Her habit of departing public transportation when she starts to have a full-blown asthma attack is one mode of environmental control: she avoids exposure by exiting an unbreathable space. But Lily also describes a second mode of controlled care. If she is unable to step off the trolley, she will try to breathe *through* her asthma. She takes a few deep breaths to try to slow down and allow her lungs to recuperate. The breath control tactics that Lily and many others use in the face of symptoms can be interpreted as a mode of making care time. Lily makes care time by slowing down, paying attention, and allowing for respiratory repair. The space of care time helps Lily to stay calm as she breathes through her attack. It is, nevertheless, a care time forced by the built environment of SEPTA. When people with asthma do not have control over environmental exposures, they often attempt to manage symptoms using different kinds of embodied engagements, some of which can be read as the creation of parallel or embedded timescapes to breathe in.

Attunement and breath control are the tactics of individual breathers who have waded into public spaces where there are no care infrastructures and minimal carescapes. During my years in Philadelphia, I have witnessed SEPTA passengers using rescue inhalers on countless occasions. Each time I share a trolley car with someone who is unable to breathe, I wonder how we might start to make the world more breathable for more people. Are there small actions, for instance, that might improve everyone's ability to breathe? For instance, could SEPTA add messaging to its communication systems to educate passengers about how certain kinds of products contribute to unbreathable atmospheres? Or could it publicize real-time air quality information at SEPTA stops? Often in discussions of care or maintenance for public infrastructures, the focus is on how to make systems more efficient, financially and temporally. What if care for infrastructures made these spaces more breathable, too? I think immediately of Halifax, Nova Scotia, a city that adopted a scent-free policy for public spaces and workplaces at the end of the twentieth century in response to a rise in environmental illnesses like asthma.[1] Policy makers in Philadelphia could help expand the city's asthma carescape by drawing more public infrastructure into the network of initiatives and organizations working to address the local epidemic.

In Philadelphia, it is very clear that asthma is produced not only through a lack of care for environment and infrastructure but also through the legacy of poverty and structural racism, conditions that require much deeper and more systematic political and economic intervention than can be provided through carefully worded SEPTA announcements. Still, I think it is important to consider the immediate, additive effects that small-scale interventions could have. This kind of thinking is needed to address complex, layered environmental health problems such as asthma and the local epidemic. Interventions are needed at multiple scales.

All of the modes of care described in this book could be read as forms of making time that engage with the breathing body, place, and environment in different ways. Some forms of care engage directly with physiology and biochemistry, using respiratory rhythms or medication adherence. Other modes of care focus on infrastructure, policy, and populations. They engage with environmental change, incorporate emerging technologies into health care systems, and focus care on such vulnerable population groups as children and the elderly. These various modes of care reflect the different timescapes through which asthma has been addressed.[2] Care is made in specific, contextual configurations that are infused with social, political, and economic relations and legacies. Through my analysis in this book, I have worked to thicken the meanings and practices of care by examining how different care practices are situated in and by "webs of care."[3] In so doing, I have aimed to contribute to existing and emerging ethical frameworks in science and technology studies and public health—both of which are highly interdisciplinary fields.[4] Such work is particularly important in the time of climate change, as new webs of nonhuman relations are shaping environmental health conditions like asthma anew, and likely making the disease and epidemic more dire.

The care practices I have documented in this book mediate interactions between the body and the environment through strategies and tactics that engage with timescapes in distinct ways—with data, the breath, policy, pharmaceuticals, and communities of practice. For example, two forms of pharmaceutical treatments, rescue inhalers and controller medications, are directed at the biochemistry of breathers, but they work at different time-scales and in different spaces. Rescue inhalers are designed to work imme-diately to open airways when breathers are experiencing symptoms; con-troller medications are intended to keep breathers' immune systems and inflammatory responses in check over time so that they never react to the environment with asthma symptoms. Controller medications work through a daily therapeutic rhythm, whereas rescue inhalers intervene during asth-matic events.

One of the defining qualities of asthma is that it disorders breathing. Yet breathing is both voluntary and involuntary. The breath is something that an individual can respond to, direct, and control. This access to embod-ied responses lends itself to specific kinds of care practices, which may or may not be seen in other disease conditions. Two forms of breath control have been described in this book—the homegrown techniques devised by asthma sufferers and the Buteyko breathing technique. Both forms engage with asthma in time and place and in ways that parallel pharmaceutical care practices that are made possible by rescue and controller medications. The timescapes of care are distinct here. One stark difference between these two forms lies in the immediacy of care for symptoms-in-the-moment and the long-term nature of chronic care infrastructures that make preventive care possible for some. My interviews with asthma sufferers revealed that many people with asthma have developed strategies that engage and direct the breathing body in the moment of attack. Breathers work with the breath to stay calm and gain control over airways run amok, and also to assess the severity of the attack itself. They develop these informal breath control tactics over time, through experiences with asthma. Such tactics are anchored in attunement, in sensing the body in place, but they are sometimes also informed by breathers' past interactions with caregivers who coached them through attacks. These breath control strategies con-stitute an ad hoc, informal mode of care in practice.

In contrast to the homegrown tactics that asthma sufferers develop through illness experience, breath control techniques may also be more formalized, such as in the case of respiratory retraining. The Buteyko method is one example of a regimented system of breath control practice. It incorporates a degree of embodied attunement to the breath but relies mostly on a rhythmic practice performed several times a day. Importantly, the technique is a living tradition of practice that is cared for (in a different way) by an international community of breathing educators. This com-munity has helped to standardize BBT as it has become more widespread as a mode of care, but it has also evolved BBT and made it more accessible to more people. Stylistically, homegrown breath control techniques and BBT are quite distinct as practices. Similar to the contrast between the rescue inhaler and controller medication, there are significant temporal and emplaced differences between homegrown breath control practices and formal respiratory retraining. The homegrown tactics of asthma sufferers, for example, are always used in response to asthma symptoms, in the event of disordered breathing, similar to the way rescue inhalers are used. They are developed through experience and attunement and are used in the context of acute illness events. By contrast, the Buteyko breathing technique is designed to stave off symptoms, reconfigure body systems, and improve the quality of life over time through a regular therapeutic practice that shifts the body's respiratory rhythms. Rather than learned strictly through experience and attunement, BBT is supported by a community of educators who use a formalized training system. The regimentation, rhythmicity, and infrastructure that support BBT constitute a system similar to the one that supports use of controller medications, which also relies on a specific kind of chronic care infrastructure in its emphasis on maintenance and prevention.

In this book I have often addressed breath control and pharmaceutical use separately to describe differences in how they are experienced and practiced as modes of care. Yet often these modes of care are bundled and used together. In part, this phenomenon reflects differences in access to and affordability of these different modes of care. Rescue inhalers are much less expensive than controller medications, and a number of those I interviewed indicated that they were taking only half the prescribed doses of their controller medications to make them last longer. Homegrown breath control techniques, of course, are developed through the illness experience, free of charge. BBT requires slightly more financial and temporal investment than homegrown techniques, but it is inexpensive in comparison to prescription asthma medications. These different modes of care also reflect different means of making and responding to time, which are entangled with various kinds of emplacements, such as access to health care, geographic region, work conditions, and living situations. Asthma has both acute and chronic valences, and its episodic character stems from the fact that it is an environmental health condition—a different kind of emplacement.

Asthma is a chronic disease condition, and many people live with this form of disordered breathing across the life course. The delivery of clinical care and pharmaceutical treatments to people with asthma, particularly people with moderate or severe forms of the disease, happens within chronic care infrastructures that create standards of practice, generate patient records, communicate information, and distribute medication. Chronic care infrastructures sink such practices as taking medication, tracking asthma control, and scheduling routine doctors' appointments into systems and networks that can support consistent disease management. These infrastructures, too, situate care practices temporally and spatially. Importantly, public health and biomedical research has repeatedly shown that consistent access to health care produces better disease outcomes.

In chapter 4, I have looked at how mobile asthma apps are using emerging digital infrastructure to extend existing health care systems. Many asthma care apps are designed to cultivate and reinforce specific kinds of care practices—such as those prescribed by medical providers—through tracking functions, notification systems, data visualizations, and online communities. Some apps, like Propeller and AHA, look beyond individual users to further researchers' understanding of population health. While it is still too early to determine what impacts care data will have on health care, researchers should pay attention to how well a given app is embedded in and extends existing chronic care infrastructures—of users, medical providers, hospitals, and insurance companies. Although these apps offer tremendous potential to draw more users into health care systems, they also raise serious questions about the quality of care.

The carescapes emerging to address asthma in an era of climate change resituate care practices at new environmental timescales. In some cases, they move beyond triggers as singular objects of concern to focus on atmospheres, built environments, and ecosystems. Although I have explicitly engaged with only one example of a carescape in this book (the pairing of the "healthy homes" curriculum with climate change education), many other responses to the contemporary asthma epidemic could be seen as contributing to growing carescapes. Local laws that prohibit vehicle idling around schools and state-level policies that allow students with asthma to carry and use their inhalers in school are just two examples. Not coincidentally, both of these responses are directed toward children and schools. Effective carescapes cannot emerge without policy implementation, and public health advocates often find more political will to implement public health policies when children's health is at stake. The Climate, Health, and Home project described in chapter 5 brought together public and private partners to conduct outreach and synthesize programming, with better results than either private or public organizations could achieve on their own. The layered engagement produced through the project's workshops connected the home environment to the local environment, as well as to public and nonprofit services. A core goal of the project was to show

how individual care practices are nested in various scapes, including care-scapes created through the workshops.[5]

Scholars can contribute to the development of carescapes by producing research that informs policy and design, supports community-based activism, and generates data that stakeholders can use. The field of science and technology studies has long embraced public engagement, but recent work has inspired a new generation of projects and conversations around "making and doing" in research.[6] To some extent, the turn toward making and doing has been situated in relation to conversations about the politics of care in research, including the ethical role of social science and humanities scholars in research and its outcomes. My role in the Climate, Health, and Home project allowed me to contribute to the development of asthma carescapes locally. I end this volume with some recommendations for the future of asthma care derived from those experiences.

This book project has made me acutely aware of the need for better ground-level public health care. Although the following recommendations may seem basic and somewhat obvious, at the time of this writing I find it crucial to reiterate foundational public health principles that have pointed the way to effective asthma care, and perhaps even prevention, for the past two decades. Making the world more breathable requires the development of more just and creative asthma carescapes that build on existing emplaced care practices and extend successful care infrastructures in ways that knit together new webs of care.

My first and most urgent recommendation is that all people be provided with routine access to high-quality medical care. Countless studies have shown that for people with asthma, lack of access to health care is associated with poor control of the disease, greater use of emergency services, and high mortality rates. Access to affordable health care not only enables asthma sufferers to obtain lifesaving medications, such as rescue inhalers, but also keeps them in contact with doctors. Regular medical care ensures that they have access to up-to-date information about the disease as well as associated care technologies, like asthma action plans, that instruct breathers how to respond when they experience symptoms. For the vast majority of people with asthma, rescue inhalers and controller medications produce drastic improvements in symptoms and quality of life. As many of my interviewees told me, not being able to breathe is terrifying. Asthma can kill you in a matter of minutes. Full stop. While some of those I interviewed expressed distrust and resentment toward pharmaceutical companies and concern about the long-term side effects of medications, almost all indicated that they want access to a rescue inhaler when symptoms arise. Although my analysis has considered contemporary

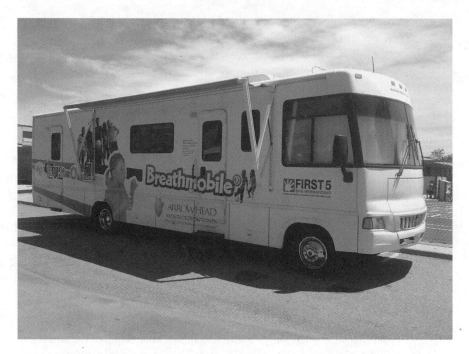

The Breathmobile is a free asthma clinic for K–12 students in San Bernardino County, California. The Breathmobile program began in Los Angeles County in 1993 and is active in nine locations across the United States. This photograph was taken during my fieldwork in May 2013.

asthma care in relation to the phenomenon of biomedicalization, which includes an overreliance on pharmaceutical interventions, this should not detract from the urgent need to make health care accessible to everyone. Inadequate access to health care is a long-standing social justice issue that is deeply entangled with the contemporary asthma epidemic.

My second recommendation echoes the hope of one of the Buteyko breathing educators quoted in chapter 3: every prescription for an inhaler should be accompanied by a breathing lesson. Respiratory retraining, including the Buteyko breathing technique, has been shown to be an effective mode of asthma care, associated with a reduction in symptoms and medication use as well as improvements in quality of life. The research presented in this book makes clear that asthma sufferers develop their own breathing techniques to care for disordered breathing, whether or not they have formal training. Sometimes people with asthma enact this mode of care before using a rescue inhaler, in an attempt to stave off the need to use medication. Others use breath control when a rescue inhaler is unavailable.

My interviews with asthma sufferers show that breath control is a gut-level response to disordered breathing, a mode of care used both when medication is on hand and when it is not. This embodied response to asthma symptoms is something that should be explored more systematically through peer-reviewed research, with the goal of developing breathing education to complement pharmaceutical treatments. Such work would be a step toward making time for a kind of care time that can operate in tandem with other timescales involved in disordered breathing and its care.

My third recommendation is that local, state, and federal governments invest in care for the built environment—homes, schools, public transportation, and other indoor breathing spaces. Some indoor environments are unbreathable through poor design, but even thoughtfully constructed spaces deteriorate over time, as materials age. Policy makers must channel more resources toward the maintenance and repair of aging twentieth-century infrastructures, as well as toward better environmental health design for infrastructures in the making.[7] In the contexts of affordable housing and disaster relief, the situation is urgent, as unstable and degraded built environments contribute to increased asthma prevalence and poor treatment outcomes. These problems are of growing concern, not only because of the difficulties of maintaining infrastructures but also because of the impacts of climate change and shifting ecological landscapes.

Finally, the United States needs to take serious action to address climate change at multiple scales and using a range of strategies. Stronger environmental regulations are needed to protect human health. The asthma epidemic has become the most clear-cut example of why we need policies that reduce air pollution and chemical exposures at multiple scales—in consumer products, small business practices, transportation systems (including roadway and vehicle design), building emissions, energy infrastructures, and industrial facilities. All of these are responsible (to varying degrees) for contributing to global climate change, and they have also been associated with respiratory diseases. Scientists have documented the connection between climate change and increased asthma prevalence as well as increased difficulty in managing the disease. Vulnerable population groups with asthma, including people living in low-income communities, children, and the elderly, are especially susceptible to the impacts of climate change.

To achieve the kind of care needed to ethically and justly address these large-scale issues, the asthma epidemic and climate change, we must make a concerted effort and employ a multitude of tactics. We need webs of care that make time for asthma care in the era of climate change.

ACKNOWLEDGMENTS

I thank my editor, Jason Weidemann, at the University of Minnesota Press, for helping cultivate this book and providing thoughtful reflection on the project over the course of several years. Gabriel Levin and Rachel Moeller were amazingly supportive in *Breathtaking*'s production, as was the entire University of Minnesota Press staff—endless thanks to this team. I am also deeply grateful to Audra Wolfe, who helped me write the material in more concrete and accessible ways in the final days of this project; I am forever a better writer for working with her. And also for working with Judy Selhorst, who copyedited the manuscript and made the text more fun to read.

This book is a spin-off of a much larger, collaborative social science study of global environmental health, The Asthma Files. Since joining the project in 2009, I have participated in a research community of more than two dozen scholars who have documented and examined together the production of air quality and its associated health effects. I am deeply grateful for the years of rich conversation on this issue and the many collaborative endeavors generated from it.Kim Fortun and Mike Fortun, who started this project more than a decade ago, have been collaborators and mentors throughout this research. I am endlessly thankful for their friendship as well as for our many years of thinking together. I thank Allison Morgan and Lindsay Poirier for their generous reading and feedback on drafts of the manuscript. Dan Price and Brandon Costelloe-Kuehn, who have also worked on The Asthma Files project, have been extraordinary collaborators as well. Tomie Hahn's early mentorship on this project has been an enduring source of wisdom and inspiration.

I conducted fieldwork at many sites over the past eight years, and this was possible only because of the generosity of many interlocutors, who opened their doors, shared their work, and told stories about their own experiences with asthma and its care. This book is indebted to them. Many thanks also to organizations that I spent time conducting fieldwork with, including United Mountain Defense in Knoxville, Tennessee; the Breathmobile programs in Oakland, Los Angeles, and San Bernardino County, California; staff members at the American Lung Association in several cities; the Buteyko Breathing Educators Association and the broader educator community; Sasha and Thomas Yakovick-Fredricksen; and the Regional Asthma Management Program in California. In Philadelphia, Russ Zerbo, Rachael Greenberg, Saleem Chapman, Richard Johnson, Jessica Caum, Julia Menzo, Deepa Mankikar, Shawana Mitchell, Andrew Goodman, and Thomas Flaherty from the Climate and Urban Systems Partnership have been amazing collaborators, and I am very grateful to have had the opportunity to work with and learn from this group over the years.

I thank Chris Kelty, Elizabeth Roberts, John Hartigan, and Tim Choy for reading early bits and pieces of writing that would eventually become *Breathtaking*. The book benefited tremendously from talks I gave in the Department of History and Sociology of Science at the University of Pennsylvania (many thanks to Ramah McKay for inviting me) and in the Department of Anthropology at the University of Michigan. A very special thanks to Elizabeth Roberts and Scott Stonington for their generative engagements with early versions of this book project.

Three colleagues in science and technology studies at Drexel University really made this book possible. Kelly Joyce was a steady and sure supporter of the project from day one. As the director of the Center for Science, Technology, and Society, she helped me in countless ways to start, continue, and finish the work. This book might not have happened without Chloe Silverman's encouragement, advice, and supply of caffeinated beverages. She is a writing partner and colleague extraordinaire. Gwen Ottinger provided inspiration, laughter, nourishment, and advice, making the writing process a lighter and more joyful experience than it would have been if I had been thinking alone. Although Vincent Duclos joined our Drexel Center at the tail end of this project, I am endlessly grateful for our robust and engaged conversations about the book and about our ongoing research.

Breathtaking was able to find footing after Ian Whitmarsh and Laura Mamo workshopped the very first draft with me; their generous, provocative reading kept me inspired until the very end. I am especially grateful to Joshua Reno and Anthony Hatch for reviewing the manuscript and providing wonderfully productive, critical, and encouraging commentary, which took the manuscript into its current form. Britt Dahlberg, Nick Shapiro, and Christy Spackman have been amazing colleagues and interlocutors over the years; the project has been shaped and instigated by our ongoing conversations. Conversations with Susan Bell, Richard Dilworth, Christian Hunold, Scott Knowles, Jake Lahne, Brent Luvaas, Mimi Sheller, Diane Sicotte, and Amy Slaton have also guided me along the way. A very special thanks to Irene Cho, Melissa Mansfield, and Sarah Saxton, whose administrative support—for myself, research assistants, and visiting colleagues—made all of this possible. And also for their friendship, nourishing conversations, and perfectly timed offers of candy and baked goods.

I thank Drexel University students Linda Croskey, Ami Diallo, Dalton George, Mel Jeske, Alex Skula, and Kerri Yandrich for helping conduct background research and preparing for interviews that shaped this book. I also thank all of the students who have worked with me through the Philadelphia Health and Environment Ethnography Lab: Eman Addish, Danielle Bartolanzo, Alexis Carlsson, Amelia Fischer, Chloe Hriso, Anna Katenta, Greg Kunkel, Matt Lesser, Cat Lowther, Daisy Manapsal, Dawn McDougall, Kathryn McNamara, Maggie McNulty, Eliza Nobles, Derek Parrott, Bhavika Patel, Shreya Patel, Hined Rafeh, Britt Salen, Lee Serpas, and Bucky Stanton. Our work together has powerfully shaped my scholarship.

My parents, Patricia and Peter Kenner, have been absolutely amazing in providing various kinds of support while I worked on this book. I have not yet been able to imagine what kind of thanks could possibly match all their care. My sisters, Christine Kenner and Amanda LaPlante, and brother-in-law, Greg LaPlante, are the best of friends and have kept me laughing, well fed, and hopeful throughout this long project. Jisela, Natalie, Christopher, and Olivia—your boundless creativity is my inspiration. Finally, to Lena, who has told me to write for as long as I can remember.

Introduction

1. At the time of this attack, Jess was thirty-four years old. He grew up in a white, working-class family from rural Appalachia, and routine medical care for his allergic asthma ended when he turned eighteen. He has never received health insurance benefits as an employee.

2. Girsh et al., "A Study on the Epidemiology of Asthma."

3. The Asthma and Allergy Foundation of America publishes an annual report that pulls together multiple data sets to compare asthma across the hundred largest metropolitan areas in the United States. For example, see Asthma and Allergy Foundation of America, *2015 Asthma Capitals*. In these rankings, Philadelphia has routinely been found to be one of the worst major cities to live in with asthma.

4. A number of anthropologists and humanities scholars have written about atmosphere, worlding, and affect in ways that have inspired this book. See, for example, Stewart, "Atmospheric Attunements"; Shapiro, "Attuning to the Chemosphere"; Fortun, "Ethnography in Late Industrialism"; Sloterdijk, *Terror from the Air*; Sloterdijk, *Bubbles*; Choy, *Ecologies of Comparison*; Górska, *Breathing Matters*.

5. Throughout this book, I use the terms *breather, asthmatic, asthma sufferer,* and *person with disordered breathing* interchangeably. Of these terms, *breather* is the most ambiguous. I borrow it from Tim Choy, who borrowed it from economists. See Choy, *Ecologies of Comparison*.

6. Celenza et al., "Thunderstorm Associated Asthma"; Wallis et al., "A Major Outbreak of Asthma."

7. Celenza et al., "Thunderstorm Associated Asthma"; Wallis et al., "A Major Outbreak of Asthma"; Dabrera et al., "Thunderstorm Asthma"; Grundstein et al., "Thunderstorm-Associated Asthma."

8. Grundstein et al., "Thunderstorm-Associated Asthma."

9. On increased allergy sensitivity related to climate change, see Schmidt, "Pollen Overload." For a more extensive treatment of this issue, see U.S. Global Change Research Program, *The Impacts of Climate Change on Human Health.*

10. Wood, "Thunderstorm Asthma."

11. Rob Nixon's idea of slow violence and Kim Fortun's discussion of late industrialism have helped me think about how the asthma epidemic is produced by outdated and failing infrastructures and policies. See Nixon, *Slow Violence and the Environmentalism of the Poor*; Fortun, "Ethnography in Late Industrialism." See also Shapiro, "Attuning to the Chemosphere."

12. Choy, *Ecologies of Comparison.*

13. Brown, *Toxic Exposures*; Kroll-Smith et al., *Illness and the Environment*; Whitmarsh, *Biomedical Ambiguity.*

14. Jackson, *Asthma.*

15. Martin et al., "The Politics of Care in Technoscience"; Puig de la Bellacasa, *Matters of Care.*

16. Reno, "Beyond Risk"; Hahn, *Sensational Knowledge.*

17. María Puig de la Bellacasa has developed the idea of "making time for care time." See Puig de la Bellacasa, "Making Time for Soil"; Puig de la Bellacasa, *Matters of Care.* Sophie Bowlby has also written about temporality in care work, and Matthew Wolf-Meyer has written about therapeutic rhythms. See Bowlby, "Recognising the Time–Space Dimensions of Care"; Wolf-Meyer, "Therapy, Remedy, Cure." All of these ideas have shaped my thinking about time in asthma care.

18. Clarke et al., *Biomedicalization*; Clarke et al., "Biomedicalization"; Bell and Figert, *Reimagining (Bio)medicalization, Pharmaceuticals, and Genetics.*

19. Trnka, *One Blue Child.*

20. Ibid.

21. Puig de la Bellacasa, *Matters of Care.*

22. Global Initiative for Asthma, *Global Strategy for Asthma Management.*

23. Gold and Wright, "Population Disparities in Asthma"; Jackson et al., "The Contributions of Allergic Sensitization"; von Mutius and Martinez, "Inconclusive Results of Randomized Trials."

24. Wenzel, "Asthma Phenotypes."

25. Quoted in Harding, "Fernando Martinez," 725.

26. "A Plea to Abandon Asthma as a Disease Concept"; Whitmarsh, *Biomedical Ambiguity.*

27. Anderson, "Endotyping Asthma," 1108. The model that Anderson refers to here is the Th2-inflammation hypothesis, which has dominated research and innovation in asthma science since the 1990s. See also Holgate, "Pathogenesis of Asthma."

28. Centers for Disease Control and Prevention, "National Health Interview Survey (NHIS) Data."

29. Moorman et al., "National Surveillance of Asthma."

30. I have found Luce Irigary's work *The Forgetting of Air in Martin Heidegger* useful for thinking about the ontological dimension of air and breathing, how the qualities of air and breathing are difficult to pin down and define.

31. Mitman, *Breathing Space.*

32. Akinbami et al., "Changing Trends in Asthma Prevalence."

33. Moorman et al., "National Surveillance of Asthma."

34. Bryant-Stephens et al., "Brief Report of a Low-Cost Street-Corner Methodology."

35. CDC data cited in Mitman, *Breathing Space,* 162.

36. Akinbami et al., "Changing Trends in Asthma Prevalence."

37. Moorman et al., "National Surveillance of Asthma."

38. Whitmarsh, *Biomedical Ambiguity.*

39. Rona, "Asthma and Poverty."

40. Rosenthal, "The Soaring Cost of a Simple Breath."

41. "Ranking Member Cummings and Chairman Sanders." Although albuterol is most often administered by inhaler, it may also be prescribed in tablet form.

42. Jena et al., "The Impact of the US Food and Drug Administration Chlorofluorocarbon Ban," 1172.

43. Rosenthal, "The Soaring Cost of a Simple Breath."

44. Ibid.

45. Callander and Schofield, "Effect of Asthma on Falling into Poverty."

46. Centers for Disease Control and Prevention, "National Health Interview Survey (NHIS) Data."

47. Centers for Disease Control and Prevention, "Vital Signs."

48. Nurmagambetov et al., "The Economic Burden of Asthma."

49. Pols, *Care at a Distance*; Mol et al., *Care in Practice.*

50. For recent reviews of the literature on care, see Martin et al., "The Politics of Care in Technoscience"; Puig de la Bellacasa, *Matters of Care.*

51. Mol, *The Logic of Care*; Mol et al., *Care in Practice.*

52. My thinking about "scales" of care has been influenced by Tim Choy's work on environmentalism in Hong Kong; see Choy, *Ecologies of Comparison.* See also Strathern, *Partial Connections.*

53. This concept of attunement is drawn from Kathleen Stewart's work on atmospheric attunement. In addition to her emphasis on the embodied, affective experience of the world, my thinking encompasses the concept of worlding—how attunement becomes a place from which to engage the world. Here Stewart draws on Nigel Thrift's work on a "geography of what happens—a speculative topography of the everyday sensibilities now consequential to living through things." Stewart, "Atmospheric Attunements," 445; Thrift, *Non-representational Theory.* For other work on attunement, see Shapiro, "Attuning to the Chemosphere"; Choy, *Ecologies of Comparison*; Anderson, "Affective Atmospheres"; Ingold, *The Life of Lines.*

54. Tomie Hahn's work has been a touchstone for my thinking about how embodiment orients and shapes responses. See Hahn, *Sensational Knowledge*. See also Hamington, *Embodied Care*.

55. The breath is more accessible, as both a voluntary and an involuntary physiological mechanism, than the medical conditions described in accounts that typically contrast control and care. On blood sugar, see Mol, *The Logic of Care*. On care ethics, see Puig de la Bellacasa, *Matters of Care*.

56. Mol, *The Logic of Care*, 39.

57. Jackson, *Asthma*; Mitman, *Breathing Space*; Whitmarsh, *Biomedical Ambiguity*.

58. Elias et al., "Airway Remodeling in Asthma"; James, "Airway Remodeling in Asthma."

59. Adam, *Timescapes of Modernity*, 9.

60. Importantly, Puig de la Bellacasa's work is geared toward displacing and disrupting "anthropocentered temporalities." I fear that, unfortunately, I reinforce them once again with my focus on breathing and asthma care, but I do work to join together ecological temporalities and respiratory ones. Puig de la Bellacasa, *Matters of Care*, 12.

61. Ibid., 23.

62. Bowker and Star, *Sorting Things Out*; Baker and Millerand, "Infrastructuring Ecology"; Langstrup, "Chronic Care Infrastructures and the Home"; Danholt and Langstrup, "Medication as Infrastructure."

63. Langstrup, "Chronic Care Infrastructures and the Home."

64. Ticktin, *Causalities of Care*; Han, *Life in Debt*; Martin et al., "The Politics of Care in Technoscience"; Puig de la Bellacasa, "Matters of Care in Technoscience"; Puig de la Bellacasa, "Making Time for Soil"; Puig de la Bellacasa, *Matters of Care*.

65. Alex Nading's work on dengue in Nicaragua and Michelle Murphy's work on sick building syndrome are two very examples of how environmental health conditions and their care become domestic. Nading, *Mosquito Trails*; Murphy, *Sick Building Syndrome*. The analysis of where care is located, in public or private domains, began with Gilligan, *In a Different Voice*.

66. Bowlby, "Recognising the Time–Space Dimensions of Care"; Ivanova et al., "Care in Place."

67. Among these are the American Lung Association's Open Airways for Schools program, initiatives by the Allergy and Asthma Foundation of America, Breathmobile clinics in cities around the United States, and the policy work conducted by the Regional Asthma Management Program in California.

68. Mol, *The Logic of Care*, 35.

69. For critical discussion of how governments care for populations, including how governmental modes of care can be oppressive and violent toward the populations they target, see Ticktin, *Causalities of Care*; Murphy, "Unsettling Care"; Han, *Life in Debt*; Stevenson, *Life beside Itself*.

70. Martin et al., "The Politics of Care in Technoscience."

71. This particular set of questions is drawn from Martin et al.'s 2015 review "The Politics of Care in Technoscience," but theories of care have been engaging with power relationships since the 1970s.

72. Gibson, *To Breathe Freely.*

73. My use of multisited ethnography for this project bears this out. Fortun, "Ethnography in/of/as Open Systems"; Marcus, "Ethnography in/of the World System"; Massey, *For Space.*

74. Martin et al., "The Politics of Care in Technoscience."

75. Murphy, *Seizing the Means of Reproduction,* 12.

76. Fortun, "Scaling and Visualizing Multi-sited Ethnography," 74. For anthropological work that addresses "scale" in methodology, see also Fortun and Fortun, "Anthropologies of the Sciences"; Choy, *Ecologies of Comparison*; Strathern, *Partial Connections.*

77. According to environmental historian Gregg Mitman, "disturbing data" on mortality, prevalence, and hospitalizations in the mid-1980s led to a state-level asthma apparatus, and the epidemic became one of the most well-known public health conditions in the 1990s. Mitman, *Breathing Space,* 245.

78. For international standards for severe asthma management, see Chung et al., "International ERS/ATS Guidelines."

79. Brody, "A Breathing Technique Offers Help."

80. See Kenner, "Asthma on the Move."

81. Clarke et al., "Biomedicalization."

82. For information on the environmental health projects I worked on in Philadelphia, see the website of the Philadelphia Health and Environment Ethnography Lab, http://www.pheel.info. In addition to the Climate, Health, and Homes project, which is documented in this volume, my research included a project on scrapyard reporting and a district-wide survey on perceptions of environmental hazards and health impacts.

83. Whitmarsh and Trnka do address everyday lived experiences in their ethnographies of asthma, but their works are much more firmly situated within and in conversation with the clinic. See Whitmarsh, "Biomedical Ambivalence"; Trnka, *One Blue Child.*

1. Attuning to Asthma in Time and Place

1. Mitman, *Breathing Space.*

2. Del Giacco et al., "Exercise and Asthma."

3. Many examples are available in Cohen's multiyear series in *Allergy and Asthma Proceedings,* "Asthma among the Famous." See also Jackson, *Asthma.*

4. Dumit, *Drugs for Life*; Greene, *Prescribing by Numbers*; Brownlee, *Overtreated.*

5. For a thorough review of the social science literature on illness normalization, see Joachim and Acorn, "Living with Chronic Illness." For a careful discussion of how normalization affects chronic disease management, see Charmaz, *Good Days, Bad Days*. Bowker and Star's classic *Sorting Things Out* has been a touchstone for thinking about the importance of classification systems and the way such systems travel between communities of practice. See also Jutel, *Putting a Name to It*.

6. Brookes, *Catching My Breath*, 12.

7. Ibid., 31.

8. The ontological questions raised by my asthmatic interlocutors remind me of the same kinds of questions, and questioned states and relationships, that Elizabeth Grosz details in *Time Travels*, in her chapter on Merleau-Ponty and Bergson. I have also found Doreen Massey's work crucial for thinking about linearity and pacing in disease. See Massey, *For Space*.

9. Stewart, "Atmospheric Attunements," 445.

10. Brookes, *Catching My Breath*, 34–35.

11. Stewart, "Atmospheric Attunements."

12. For examples of recent work on the definition of asthma, see Fitzpatrick et al., "Heterogeneity of Severe Asthma in Childhood"; Bel et al., "Diagnosis and Definition of Severe Refractory Asthma"; Moore et al., "Identification of Asthma Phenotypes"; Lötvall et al., "Asthma Endotypes."

13. Global Initiative for Asthma, *Global Strategy for Asthma Management*, 14.

14. Ibid.

15. Ibid., 15.

16. See Lockey, "Defining Phenotypes."

17. Wenzel, "Asthma Phenotypes," 716.

18. Ibid.

19. On cultural representations of asthma and how they shape patient perspectives, see Clark, "Asthma Episodes." For a review of how negative patient perceptions create barriers to disease management, see Ahmad and Ismail, "Stigma in the Lives of Asthma Patients."

20. Kenner, "The Healthy Asthmatic."

21. Wenzel, "Asthma Phenotypes."

22. A number of excellent histories of asthma describe the role played by immunology in the conceptualization and treatment of asthma in the nineteenth and twentieth centuries. See Jackson, *Asthma*; Mitman, *Breathing Space*; Keirns, "Better Than Nature."

23. Melgert et al., "Are There Reasons Why Adult Asthma Is More Common in Females?"; Bel, "Another Piece to the Puzzle"; Siroux et al., "Phenotypic Determinants of Uncontrolled Asthma."

24. See Lockey, "Defining Phenotypes."

25. Dr. Francis Rackemann, an allergist who studied asthma for more than four decades, published a number of papers in the 1940s that suggested different

classifications of the disease, such as a theory of external versus internal asthma. His theory incorporated age of disease onset and distinguished allergic asthma from other kinds. It is unclear how widely Rackemann's work may have been taken up in general practice. See, for example, Rackemann, "A Working Classification of Asthma"; Rackemann, "Intrinsic Asthma." See also Diamant et al., "Summing Up 100 Years of Asthma."

26. Reddel, "An Official American Thoracic Society/European Respiratory Society Statement."

27. Global Initiative for Asthma, *Global Strategy for Asthma Management*; National Asthma Education and Prevention Program, *Expert Panel Report 3*; Reddel, "An Official American Thoracic Society/European Respiratory Society Statement."

28. Global Initiative for Asthma, *Global Strategy for Asthma Management*, 15.

29. Ibid., 16.

30. Ibid., 18.

31. Ibid., 17.

32. Although spirometers are the recommended means of assessing airflow limitation for asthma, these machines are rarely present in general practice settings, where asthma is frequently diagnosed. Furthermore, while the National Asthma Education and Prevention Program has identified spirometry as "an essential objective measure to establish the diagnosis of asthma," historian of medicine Lundy Braun has shown otherwise, and there is resounding clinical evidence that challenges the relationship between asthma and respiratory function as measured by both spirometry and peak flow meters. National Asthma Education and Prevention Program, *Expert Panel Report 3*, 11; Braun, *Breathing Race into the Machine*. See also Eng et al., "Testing Spirometers."

33. Good, *Medicine, Rationality, and Experience*; Canguillem, *On the Normal and the Pathological*.

34. Massey, reading de Certeau, describes the struggle of writing narrative in *For Space*, 25.

35. Mitman, *Breathing Space*.

36. Braman, "The Global Burden of Asthma"; Gerritsen et al., "Prognosis of Asthma from Childhood to Adulthood"; Martin et al., "Asthma from Childhood at Age 21."

37. Global Initiative for Asthma, *Global Strategy for Asthma Management*, 26.

38. Stein and Martinez, "Asthma Phenotypes in Childhood."

39. For scholarship on the work that expert patients undertake in various contexts, see Pols, "Knowing Patients"; Klawiter, *The Biopolitics of Breast Cancer*; Dumit, *Drugs for Life*; Epstein, *Impure Science*; Kroll-Smith et al., *Illness and the Environment*; Brown, *Toxic Exposures*; Mol, *The Logic of Care*; Murphy, *Sick Building Syndrome*. For a discussion of the expert patient in the context of disordered breathing, see Boulet, "The Expert Patient and Chronic Respiratory Diseases."

40. Brookes, *Catching My Breath*, 7.

41. Omalizumab is a targeted asthma treatment prescribed for allergic asthmatics over the age of twelve who have severe asthma. Darveaux and Busse have referred to it as a "biological agent," the only one currently approved for asthma treatment. Darveaux and Busse, "Biologics in Asthma."

2. Three Modes of Control as Asthma Care

1. Two examples of such advocacy organizations are the National Asthma Control Initiative and the Allergy and Asthma Foundation of America.

2. Dumit, *Drugs for Life*.

3. Global Initiative for Asthma, *Global Strategy for Asthma Management*, 26.

4. Ibid., 31.

5. Both the 2009 joint ATS/ERS statement and the GINA report note that the definition of exacerbation—as well as use of the term in clinical settings—is quite loose and needs to be better standardized for both treatment and research purposes. Reddel et al., "An Official American Thoracic Society/European Respiratory Society Statement"; Global Initiative for Asthma, *Global Strategy for Asthma Management*.

6. Global Initiative for Asthma, *Global Strategy for Asthma Management*, 31.

7. Wenzel, "Asthma Phenotypes"; Global Initiative for Asthma, *Global Strategy for Asthma Management*.

8. Global Initiative for Asthma, *Global Strategy for Asthma Management*, 26.

9. Dumit, *Drugs for Life*.

10. Reddel et al., "An Official American Thoracic Society/European Respiratory Society Statement," 65.

11. Nurmagambetov et al., "The Economic Burden of Asthma."

12. Information on the history of the National Asthma Education and Prevention Program is available on the NHLBI website, https://www.nhlbi.nih.gov.

13. National Asthma Education and Prevention Program, *Expert Panel Report 3*.

14. Information about NACI and the six action items is available on the NHLBI website, https://www.nhlbi.nih.gov.

15. The list includes everyone except stakeholders in the pharmaceutical industry; NACI's framework is anchored in pharmaceutical interests.

16. Dumit, *Drugs for Life*.

17. Braun, *Breathing Race into the Machine*.

18. Caffeine works on the body in ways similar to bronchodilators.

19. Global Initiative for Asthma, *Global Strategy for Asthma Management*, 26.

20. Brookes, *Catching My Breath*.

21. Global Initiative for Asthma, *Global Strategy for Asthma Management*, 26.

22. This is essentially what GINA recommends as a "Step 1" approach in asthma treatment. Global Initiative for Asthma, *Global Strategy for Asthma Management*.

23. Ibid., 41, 42.

24. Reddel et al., "An Official American Thoracic Society/European Respiratory Society Statement," 66.

25. Latour, "How to Talk about the Body?," 205.

26. Mol, *The Logic of Care*.

27. Pink, "From Embodiment to Emplacement."

28. Englund, "Ethnography after Globalism," 263.

29. Reno, "Beyond Risk," 517.

30. Trnka, *One Blue Child*; Pink, "From Embodiment to Emplacement."

31. Nancy Chen, for example, describes how qigong breathing exercises work to transform the mind and body to support good health. Embodied qigong practices that utilize the breath cultivate the self; sometimes these exercises also include visualization techniques. In qigong, self-cultivation and mastery of the breath allow individuals to transcend ordinary, everyday experience. Chen, *Breathing Spaces*.

32. Maynard, "Controlling Death—Compromising Life," 214.

33. Foucault, *The Birth of the Clinic*; Foucault, *Power/Knowledge*; Canguilhem, *On the Normal and the Pathological*; Maynard, "Controlling Death—Compromising Life."

34. Fortun, "Scaling and Visualizing Multi-sited Ethnography."

35. Ticktin, *Casualties of Care*; Stevenson, *Life beside Itself*; Murphy, *Seizing the Means of Reproduction*; Han, *Life in Debt*.

36. Mol, *The Logic of Care*.

37. Cynthia's home reminded me of the controlled indoor spaces used in the care of people with environmental sensitivities, in which any material objects that could trigger symptoms have been eliminated. For discussion of how such practices work in relation to different examples of environmental sensitivities, see Mitman, *Breathing Space*; Chen, *Animacies*; Brant, "Scenting a Subject"; Anderson, "Affective Atmospheres."

38. In 2013 and 2014, I made several trips to observe asthma care on one of the Breathmobiles in Southern California. During these visits, I watched as medical staff spoke extensively with parents of asthmatic children and asthma patients about triggers in their home and local environments.

39. Mitman, *Breathing Space*; Whitmarsh, *Biomedical Ambiguity*; Jackson, *Asthma*; Trnka, *One Blue Child*.

3. Counting on Breath

1. The title of this March 2010 event, held by the Buteyko Center USA (now the Breathing Center), was the "Natural Asthma Cure Workshop." Since that time, references to "cure" have been dropped from the materials on the organization's

website, replaced by discussion of "therapy" and "treatment." I have not spoken with any representatives of the center about the change in terminology, but I would surmise that it was made to protect the organization's credibility. Asthma is widely regarded as an incurable condition; any claim to the contrary invites skepticism.

2. Wenzel, "Asthma Phenotypes"; Wener and Bel, "Severe Refractory Asthma."

3. Drawing on the case of sleep disorders in the United States, Matthew Wolf-Meyer has argued that therapies—pharmaceutical, prosthetic, and behavioral—can be understood as rhythmic interventions that structure everyday lives through spatiotemporal dynamics. Wolf-Meyer, "Therapy, Remedy, Cure."

4. Lefebvre, *Rhythmanalysis*.

5. Munn, "The Cultural Anthropology of Time"; Adam, *Timescapes of Modernity*; Puig de la Bellacasa, "Making Time for Soil"; Whipp et al., *Making Time*.

6. Vuckovic, "Fast Relief"; Berlant, "Risky Bigness."

7. Adam, *Timescapes of Modernity*.

8. Puig de la Bellacasa, "Making Time for Soil," 695.

9. For in-depth discussions of time in relation to capitalism, see Adam, *Timescapes of Modernity*; Puig de la Bellacasa, *Matters of Care*; Adams et al., "Anticipation." For discussion of time in relation to health and medicine, see Vuckovic, "Fast Relief"; Berlant, "Risky Bigness"; Sanz, "Out-of-Sync Cancer Care"; Good, "The Medical Imaginary and the Biotechnical Embrace."

10. While Puig de la Bellacasa's work on care time is specifically concerned with human–nonhuman webs of care, my case study—breathing practices—does not engage the nonhuman dimensions of living and caring. Nevertheless, decentering anthropocentrism is a crucial part of Puig de la Bellacasa's theory of care, and I feel it is important to mention that this chapter does not build on her work in that specific way.

11. Buteyko, "Interview with K. P. Buteyko."

12. Puig de la Bellacasa, "Making Time for Soil," 705.

13. Buteyko, "Interview with K. P. Buteyko," n.p.

14. Clarke et al., "Biomedicalization"; Puig de la Bellacasa, "Making Time for Soil."

15. In this chapter, I situate breathing as a mundane, everyday process that needs to be cared for and is cared for through BBT. This includes the breathing practices that individuals undertake on their own as well as the group and one-on-one work that some educators and trainers do with students to support the community of practice. Many feminist scholars have addressed the significance of ordinary, everyday activities. For foundational work, see Brown and Gilligan, *Meeting at the Crossroads*; Tronto, *Moral Boundaries*; Kittay, "Taking Dependency Seriously." For more recent work, see Mol, *The Logic of Care*; Mol et al., *Care in Practice*; Martin et al., "The Politics of Care in Technoscience"; Puig de la Bellacasa, *Matters of Care*.

16. Mol, *The Logic of Care*; Mol et al., *Care in Practice*.

17. Buteyko, "Interview with K. P. Buteyko," n.p.

18. Ibid. Buteyko's accounts and use of language should be read in relation to more extensive treatments of twentieth-century Soviet science. The only available biographical information on Buteyko is told from his perspective. Given that he was conducting this research during the 1950s and 1960s, when Soviet scientists faced many political pressures, including in regard to the content of their work, his version of events should be read in relation to Soviet political culture. For an introduction to science in the Soviet Union, see Graham, *Science in Russia and the Soviet Union*.

19. Buteyko, "Interview with K. P. Buteyko," n.p.

20. There is a small body of peer-reviewed literature on BBT, and in recent years it has grown. For early work, see Cooper et al., "Effect of Two Breathing Exercises"; Bowler et al., "Buteyko Breathing Techniques in Asthma"; Opat et al., "A Clinical Trial of the Buteyko Breathing Technique"; Cowie et al., "A Randomised Controlled Trial of the Buteyko Technique"; McHugh et al., "Buteyko Breathing Technique for Asthma"; Bruton and Lewith, "The Buteyko Breathing Technique for Asthma"; Ram et al., "Breathing Retraining for Asthma." For more recent work, see Prem et al., "Comparison of the Effects of Buteyko and Pranayama Breathing Techniques"; Prasanna et al., "Effect of Buteyko Breathing Exercise"; Hassan et al., "Effect of Buteyko Breathing Technique"; Bruton and Thomas, "The Role of Breathing Training in Asthma Management."

21. Many books on the Buteyko method provide in-depth anatomical and physiological descriptions of respiration and its relationship with other biological systems. See, for example, McKeown, *Close Your Mouth*; Stark and Stark, *The Buteyko Method*; Graham, *Relief from Snoring and Sleep Apnoea*; Novozhilov, *Living without Asthma*.

22. Buteyko, "Interview with K. P. Buteyko," n.p.

23. Ibid.

24. There is some research to suggest that vital signs, and respiratory rate in particular, may be overlooked in various medical settings. See Cretikos et al., "Respiratory Rate"; Van Leuvan and Mitchell, "Missed Opportunities?"

25. Buteyko, "Interview with K. P. Buteyko," n.p.

26. Trnka, *One Blue Child*.

27. McKeown, *Close Your Mouth*; Stark and Stark, *The Buteyko Method*.

28. Altukhov, "Doctor Buteyko's Discovery Trilogy."

29. Lefebvre, *Rhythmanalysis*.

30. Steven Epstein has examined lay expertise in scientific contexts, with a focus on HIV/AIDS activism; see Epstein, *Impure Science*. On embodied health movements and their engagement with science, see Brown et al., "The Health Politics of Asthma."

31. The traditional approach is described in both McKeown, *Close Your Mouth*; and Stark and Stark, *The Buteyko Method*. Mouth taping is simply putting a piece of tape vertically across the mouth to help encourage nose breathing. Most Buteyko books and websites describe the process in further detail.

32. The vast majority of BBEs I have met at the annual meetings of the BBEA, as well as those interviewed for this study, are white and middle-class or working-class. They range in age from thirty to sixty-five. Women make up the majority of the BBE community.

33. Brody, "A Breathing Technique Offers Help."

34. These practices have been associated with pharmaceuticalization, but historical accounts of asthma, including biographies of asthmatics, suggest that a wide range of therapeutic practices are common, with asthmatics often operating in a mode of trial-and-error experimentation. On pharmaceuticalization, see Bell and Figert, *Reimagining (Bio)Medicalization, Pharmaceuticals, and Genetics*. For historical accounts of therapeutic practices, see Jackson, *Asthma*; Mitman, *Breathing Space*; Keirns, "Better Than Nature." It should also be noted that since the time of Brody's article, the pharmaceutical options for asthma treatment have widened. See, for example, Global Initiative for Asthma, *Global Strategy for Asthma Management*.

35. Dumit, *Drugs for Life*.

36. Jackson, "Asthma, Illness, and Identity": Jackson, *Asthma*. See also Cohen's series "Asthma among the Famous."

37. Jackson, *Asthma*, 9.

38. I have often wondered if Proust, like those asthmatics interviewed for this project, might have developed a series of attunement practices and his own breathing techniques. In his biography of asthma, Jackson describes Proust's suffering and quality of life but does not get into the details of how his care was enacted. Ibid.

39. Numerous studies suggest that 5 to 10 percent of asthmatics suffer from a form of the disease resistant to available treatments, increasingly referred to as refractory-resistant asthma. This form of asthma is found across severity levels, but it is concentrated among those with the most severe forms of the disease. As Kian Fan Chung writes, "In a study of the effect of combined treatment with a long-acting β-adrenergic agonist and an inhaled corticosteroid, asthma control (defined by GINA guidelines) was achieved in only 68 percent of patients with varying severity of disease, with the least number in the most severe group, suggesting that even treatment at the maximum doses allowable is not effective in all patients with asthma." Chung, "New Treatments for Severe Treatment-Resistant Asthma," 639. See also Bateman et al., "Can Guideline-Defined Asthma Control Be Achieved?"; Chung et al., "Difficult/Therapy-Resistant Asthma"; American Thoracic Society, "Proceedings of the ATS Workshop on Refractory Asthma."

40. Brody, "A Breathing Technique Offers Help." BBT is also recommended in guidelines published by the British Thoracic Society and Scottish Intercollegiate Guidelines Network, and by the U.S. Agency for Healthcare Research and Quality. See British Thoracic Society and Scottish Intercollegiate Guidelines Network, *British Guideline on the Management of Asthma*; O'Connor et al., *Breathing Exercises and/or Retraining Techniques*.

41. Medical sociologists have described and theorized how lay experts, patient and caregiver groups, and practitioner communities have mobilized to bring attention and action to marginalized treatments. See, for example, Brown et al., "The Health Politics of Asthma"; Epstein, *Impure Science*. In many cases, such movements have included strategic use of the news media. More recently, Scott Frickel and his colleagues have written about how social movements call attention to "undone science." Frickel et al., "Undone Science," 2010. See also Hess, "Medical Modernisation."

42. Orthodontists and maxillofacial surgeons also constitute an emerging audience, since these professionals are interested in combating mouth breathing, which contributes to dental problems.

43. In addition to the scholarship on undone science cited in note 39 above, the work of Adele Clarke and her colleagues on biomedicalization has helped me think through why the Buteyko tradition has been stymied in the United States. See Clarke et al., "Biomedicalization."

44. Burgess et al., "Systematic Review of the Effectiveness of Breathing Retraining."

45. Wolf-Meyer, "Therapy, Remedy, Cure," 145.

4. The Datafication of Care

1. Ruckenstein and Schüll, "The Datafication of Health," 262.

2. Propeller Health, *What Is Propeller?*, emphasis added.

3. For recent work on how environmental sensing technology may be shifting the politics of eco-management and daily human–nonhuman engagements, see Gabrys, *Program Earth*.

4. Freifeld et al., "Participatory Epidemiology."

5. Ibid., 5.

6. Ibid., 3.

7. Quoted in Smith, "Researcher Uses GPS to Find Asthma Causes."

8. See, for example, Van Sickle and Wright, "Navajo Perceptions of Asthma"; Wind et al., "Health, Place and Childhood Asthma"; Van Sickle, "Diagnosis and Management of Asthma."

9. "Discover the Gadgets That Are Improving Treatments for Asthma."

10. Mol, *The Logic of Care*.

11. See Kenner, "Asthma on the Move."

12. Langstrup, "Chronic Care Infrastructures and the Home," 1010.

13. I use pseudonyms here for the developer and his wife, as well as for the app.

14. I conducted formal interviews with nine people who worked to develop asthma care apps. These included doctors and software developers, but more than half were neither medical nor technical experts. Five of these interviews were conducted with marketing or sales representatives for the organizations developing the asthma care apps. This set of interviews took place in 2013.

15. Asthma Ally was developed by OSIA Medical, a medical technology company based in Utah.

16. For more information on AsthmaMD, see the product website, http://www.asthmamd.org.

17. Mol, *The Logic of Care*.

18. Bowker and Star, *Sorting Things Out*.

19. Both pharmaceuticalization and datafication depend on an element of trust on the part of users. See van Dijck and Poell, "Understanding the Promises and Premises of Online Health Platforms."

20. Schüll, "Data for Life," 318.

21. Mol, *The Logic of Care*.

22. App use typically drops off several months after the initial download. See Zhao et al., "Can Mobile Phone Apps Influence People's Health Behavior Change?"; Chan et al., "The Asthma Mobile Health Study"; Lane et al., "Online Recruitment Methods."

23. Apple, Inc., "Apple Introduces ResearchKit."

24. The untitled video is available on the ResearchKit website, https://www.apple.com/researchkit.

25. Icahn School of Medicine at Mount Sinai, "Asthma Mobile Health Study," accessed March 13, 2018, http://apps.icahn.mssm.edu/asthma.

26. Chan et al., "The Asthma Mobile Health Study."

27. Ibid., 360.

28. Ibid.

29. Icahn School of Medicine, *Asthma Health App, U.S. Participants*.

30. Icahn School of Medicine at Mount Sinai, "Asthma Mobile Health Study: Participant Stories," accessed March 13, 2018, http://apps.icahn.mssm.edu/asthma. All the AHA testimonials quoted in this chapter are found on this site.

31. Chan et al., "The Asthma Mobile Health Study," 360.

32. Wolf-Meyer, "Therapy, Remedy, Cure."

33. Natanson, "Digital Therapeutics."

34. Propeller's success is documented extensively in the "Press" section of the Propeller Health website, https://www.propellerhealth.com.

35. See the list of peer-reviewed publications on Propeller in the "Published Research" section of Propeller Health's website, https://www.propellerhealth.com/enterprise.

36. Propeller Health, "Louisville Data Findings."

37. Propeller Health, "Asthmapolis Relaunches as Propeller Health."

38. Propeller Health, *Live Your Life without Limits*.

39. Su et al., "Feasibility of Deploying Inhaler Sensors," 260.

40. Comstock, "Three Lessons Propeller Learned."

41. Propeller Health, "Propeller Health Receives FDA Clearance."

42. Quoted in ibid.

5. Public Health Carescapes for Climate Change

1. For recent public health studies on these factors, see Milligan et al. "Asthma in Urban Children"; Callander and Schofield, "Effect of Asthma on Falling into Poverty"; Keet et al., "Neighborhood Poverty, Urban Residence." For a historical perspective, see Mitman, *Breathing Space.*

2. The 2011–13 data on prevalence rates in Philadelphia are from Pennsylvania Department of Public Health, *2015 Asthma Prevalence Report.* National prevalence rates, which were updated in 2015, come from Centers for Disease Control and Prevention, "Asthma: Data, Statistics, and Surveillance."

3. Philadelphia Department of Public Health, *Community Health Assessment.*

4. See, for example, Alexander and Currie, "Is It Who You Are or Where You Live?"; Feyler, "The Impact of Housing Quality"; Lang and Polansky, "Patterns of Asthma Mortality in Philadelphia."

5. For more on the Healthy Rowhouse Project, see the project's website, http://healthyrowhouse.org. For more on Philly Thrive, visit http://www.philly thrive.org.

6. See Bowlby, "Recognising the Time–Space Dimensions of Care"; Ivanova et al., "Care in Place."

7. Martin et al., "The Politics of Care in Technoscience"; Atkinson-Graham et al., "Care in Context."

8. Quotations from workshop participants in this chapter are taken from my field notes and the field notes of students who conducted participant observation at the workshops. Unlike quotations in previous chapters, which are taken from formally recorded interviews, those in this chapter were not recorded in interview sessions unless indicated in the text.

9. Asthma and Allergy Foundation of America, *2015 Asthma Capitals.*

10. See the city of Philadelphia's resource and services map at http://gsg.phila .gov/map#id=b091d039d3d2495dbe02914d3216db8b.

11. "Excessive Heat, Air Quality 'Code Orange' Warning Issued."

12. The EPA archives all outdoor air quality data on its website, https://www .epa.gov, which enables users to generate reports by year and geographic location. More information about the AQI can be found in reports available in the site's "Outdoor Air Quality Data" section.

13. For more about CUSP, see the project's website, http://www.cuspproject .org.

14. The project and its resources are documented on the Philadelphia Health and Environment Ethnography Lab's website, http://www.pheel.info.

15. Bowlby, "Recognising the Time–Space Dimensions of Care," 2110.

16. Kittay, *Love's Labor.*

17. Since the 1960s, citywide air pollution may have improved in the city of Philadelphia at the scale tracked by Clean Air Act mandates, but there is good reason to suspect that improvements have been uneven across neighborhoods and planning

districts. While academic, governmental, and nongovernmental air-monitoring projects have shown that some forms of air pollution are greater around the South Philadelphia oil refinery, the ports, and the industrial facilities in the River Wards, as well as along the I-95 corridor, ethnographic research suggests that development-related air pollution is also a problem and has had greater impacts on some people than on others. Construction dust is routinely mentioned by participants in community meetings in the River Wards planning district, for example.

18. For a snapshot of construction in Center City, see Romero, "Mapping the 29 High-Rises under Construction in Philly Right Now." For insights into how people experiencing homelessness have been displaced by construction projects in Philadelphia, see Orso, "Why You're Seeing More Homelessness."

19. It should be noted that several methodological factors played into this difference. First, the structure of the earlier asthma care interviews was different from the oral history format used in the 2017 interviews. In the interviews with Philadelphia seniors, we often asked questions about environmental change relatively early, whereas in the asthma care interviews, questions about environment and place often came at the ends of the interviews. Additionally, the places differed. My interviews about asthma care practices were mostly conducted with people who lived and grew up in small towns and cities. As the fifth-largest city in the United States, and a city with a 27 percent poverty rate, Philadelphia provided quite a different landscape. Finally, while the asthma care interviews were conducted with white working- and middle-class people in their twenties, thirties, and forties, the Climate, Health, and Home interviews were conducted with African Americans in their sixties, seventies, and eighties.

20. See, for example, Brown et al., "The Health Politics of Asthma"; Krieger et al., "The Seattle–King County Healthy Homes Project"; Maantay, "Asthma and Air Pollution in the Bronx"; Loh and Sugerman-Brozan, "Environmental Justice Organizing for Environmental Health"; Corburn, *Street Science.*

21. U.S. Global Change Research Program, *The Impacts of Climate Change on Human Health.*

22. Ibid., 79.

23. Although the earliest thunderstorm asthma events were documented in 1983, the topic has received increasing attention over the past decade, especially in the past few years, as researchers have recognized the phenomenon's connection to climate change. For more on the mechanisms of thunderstorm asthma, see D'Amato et al., "Thunderstorm-Asthma and Pollen Allergy."

24. For more information on the Climate and Health Program, including resources and activities, see the CDC's website, https://www.cdc.gov.

25. The Public Health Institute is a California-based nonprofit organization that supports public health projects at various scales—local, state, national, and even international. See Public Health Institute, "PHI's Center for Climate Change and Health."

26. U.S. Global Change Research Program, *The Impacts of Climate Change on Human Health*, 72. This was one of the key findings of the USGCRP report, which was published eighteen months after the described workshop.

27. Ibid., 79.

28. For detailed social science accounts of such research, see Whitmarsh, *Biomedical Ambiguity*; Mitman, *Breathing Space*.

29. U.S. Global Change Research Program, *The Impacts of Climate Change on Human Health*, 81.

30. For more information on the EPA's Air Quality Index, see the AirNow website, https://www.airnow.gov.

31. American Public Health Association, "Community Health Workers."

32. Kruse, *Lead Hazard Control and Healthy Homes*.

33. National Asthma Education and Prevention Program, *Expert Panel Report 3*.

34. For a critique of environmental campaigns and their disconnect from people's everyday lives and concerns, see Meyer, *Engaging the Everyday*.

35. For two such accounts, see Strauss, "Girl Dies after Getting Sick at School"; Malfitano, "Philadelphia Dismissed from Lawsuit."

36. In 2004, the state of Pennsylvania passed a law stating that children can have access to and use asthma inhalers in school. As of 2011, students attending schools in the School District of Philadelphia were allowed to carry and use their inhalers in school. School District of Philadelphia, *Use of Medications/Medical Technology*. Media reports on Laporshia's death did not mention whether she had an inhaler on the day she died or whether she was allowed to use it, only that there was no nurse present.

37. Bryant-Stephens et al., "Brief Report of a Low-Cost Street-Corner Methodology."

38. These findings join those of other studies that have shown that as many as 40 percent of children living in deep poverty have asthma but are often undiagnosed and untreated. McLean et al., "Asthma among Homeless Children."

39. Bryant-Stephens et al., "Home Visits Are Needed to Address Asthma," 1526.

40. Denvir, "Philly School District Blocks a Federal Study," n.p.

41. During my fieldwork, people I spoke with would occasionally mention an environment-related school closing. It was not until one of my informants sent me an article about the NIOSH study that I started to grasp the depth of the issue. See ibid. Mentions of the NIOSH study are scattered among various documents, but I found no news reports about the study other than Denvir's. See Howard, "NIOSH and Schools"; Cox-Ganser et al., "Asthma and Asthma Symptoms in Teachers." Jerry Roseman, director of environmental science and occupational safety and health for the Philadelphia Federation of Teachers Health and Welfare Fund, has written extensively on these issues. See, for example, Roseman, "Can We Make Philadelphia Schools Safer?"; Roseman, "A Matter of Health and Safety."

42. "Philadelphia's Dirty Schools."
43. Windle, "District Scrambling to Remove Mold."
44. Nixon, *Slow Violence and the Environmentalism of the Poor*, 2.
45. Knowles, "Learning from Disaster?"

Conclusion

1. For ethnographic work on environmental sensitivities in Halifax, see Fletcher, "Environmental Sensitivity." For a brief summary of Halifax's initiation of voluntary fragrance-free policies, see Bjorn, "Halifax Celebrates 20 Years Fragrance Free."

2. Choy, *Ecologies of Comparison*; Fortun, "Scaling and Visualizing Multi-sited Ethnography"; Adam, *Timescapes of Modernity*; Strathern, *Partial Connections*.

3. See the commentary on Joan Tronto's work in Puig de la Bellacasa, *Matters of Care*.

4. Ibid.

5. Kittay, *Love's Labor*; Tronto, "Beyond Gender Difference to a Theory of Care"; Puig de la Bellacasa, *Matters of Care*.

6. For an overview of the making and doing movement, see Downey and Zuiderent-Jerak, "Making and Doing."

7. For discussion of how a lack of care for infrastructure can have negative impacts on health, see Fortun, "Ethnography in Late Industrialism"; Shapiro, "Attuning to the Chemosphere"; Murphy, *Sick Building Syndrome*; Rao et al., "Characterization of Airborne Molds, Endotoxins, and Glucans."

Adam, Barbara. *Timescapes of Modernity: The Environment and Invisible Hazards*. New York: Routledge, 1998.

Adams, Vincanne, Michelle Murphy, and Adele E. Clarke. "Anticipation: Technoscience, Life, Affect, Temporality." *Subjectivity* 28, no. 1 (2009): 246–65.

Ahmad, Sohail, and Nahlah E. Ismail. "Stigma in the Lives of Asthma Patients: A Review from the Literature." *International Journal of Pharmacy and Pharmaceutical Sciences* 7, no. 7 (2015): 40–46.

Akinbami, Lara J., Alan E. Simon, and Lauren M. Rossen. "Changing Trends in Asthma Prevalence among Children." *Pediatrics* 137, no. 1 (2015). doi:10.1542/pcds.2015-2354.

Alexander, Diane, and Janet Currie. "Is It Who You Are or Where You Live? Residential Segregation and Racial Gaps in Childhood Asthma." *Journal of Health Economics* 55 (2017): 186–200.

Altukhov, Sergey. "Doctor Buteyko's Discovery Trilogy." Last modified 2017. http://www.doctorbuteykodiscoverytrilogy.com.

American Public Health Association. "Community Health Workers." Accessed February 26, 2018. https://www.apha.org.

American Thoracic Society. "Proceedings of the ATS Workshop on Refractory Asthma: Current Understanding, Recommendations, and Unanswered Questions." *American Journal of Respiratory and Critical Care Medicine* 162, no. 6 (2000): 2341–51.

Anderson, Ben. "Affective Atmospheres." *Emotion, Space and Society* 2, no. 2 (2009): 77–81.

Anderson, Gary P. "Endotyping Asthma: New Insights into Key Pathogenic Mechanisms in a Complex, Heterogeneous Disease." *The Lancet* 372, no. 9643 (2008): 1107–19.

Apple, Inc. "Apple Introduces ResearchKit, Giving Medical Researchers the Tools to Revolutionize Medical Studies." Press release, March 9, 2015. https://www.apple.com/newsroom.

Asthma and Allergy Foundation of America. *2015 Asthma Capitals.* Landover, Md.: AAFA, 2015. http://www.aafa.org.

Atkinson-Graham, Melissa, Martha Kenney, Kelly Ladd, Cameron Michael Murray, and Emily Astra-Jean Simmonds. "Care in Context: Becoming an STS Researcher." *Social Studies of Science* 45, no. 5 (2015): 738–48.

Baker, Karen S., and Florence Millerand. "Infrastructuring Ecology: Challenges in Achieving Data Sharing." In *Collaboration in the New Life Sciences,* edited by John N. Parker, Niki Vermeulen, and Bart Penders, 111–39. London: Routledge, 2010.

Bateman, Eric D., Homer A. Boushey, Jean Bousquet, William W. Busse, Tim J. H. Clark, Romain A. Pauwels, and Søren E. Pedersen. "Can Guideline-Defined Asthma Control Be Achieved? The Gaining Optimal Asthma Control Study." *American Journal of Respiratory and Critical Care Medicine* 170, no. 8 (2004): 836–44.

Bel, Elisabeth H. "Another Piece to the Puzzle of the 'Obese Female Asthma' Phenotype." *American Journal of Respiratory and Critical Care Medicine* 188, no. 3 (2013): 263–64.

Bel, Elisabeth H., Ana Sousa, Louise Fleming, Andrew Bush, K. Fan Chung, Jennifer Versnel, Ariane H. Wagener, Scott S. Wagers, Peter J. Sterk, and Chris H. Compton. "Diagnosis and Definition of Severe Refractory Asthma: An International Consensus Statement from the Innovative Medicine Initiative (IMI)." *Thorax* 66, no. 10 (2011): 910–17.

Bell, Susan, and Anne E. Figert. *Reimagining (Bio)Medicalization, Pharmaceuticals, and Genetics: Old Critiques and New Engagements.* New York: Routledge, 2015.

Berlant, Lauren. "Risky Bigness: On Obesity, Eating, and the Ambiguity of 'Health.'" In *Against Health: How Health Became the New Morality,* edited by Jonathan M. Metzl and Anna Kirkland, 26–39. New York: New York University Press, 2010.

Bjorn, Genevieve. "Halifax Celebrates 20 Years Fragrance Free." *Daily Smell,* January 15, 2011. http://dev.thedailysmell.com.

Boulet, Louis-Philippe. "The Expert Patient and Chronic Respiratory Diseases." *Canadian Respiratory Journal* 2016 (2016). doi:10.1155/2016/9454506.

Bowker, Geoffrey C., and Susan Leigh Star. *Sorting Things Out: Classification and Its Consequences.* Cambridge, Mass.: MIT Press, 1999.

Bowlby, Sophie. "Recognising the Time–Space Dimensions of Care: Caringscapes and Carescapes." *Environment and Planning A* 44, no. 9 (2012): 2101–18.

Bowler, Simon D., Amanda Green, and Charles A. Mitchell. "Buteyko Breathing Techniques in Asthma: A Blinded Randomised Controlled Trial." *Medical Journal of Australia* 169 (1998): 575–78.

Braman, Sidney S. "The Global Burden of Asthma." Supplement, *Chest* 130, no. 1 (2006): 4S–12S.

Brant, Clare. "Scenting a Subject: Odour Poetics and the Politics of Space." *Ethnos* 73, no. 4 (2008): 544–63.

Braun, Lundy. *Breathing Race into the Machine: The Surprising Career of the Spirometer from Plantation to Genetics.* Minneapolis: University of Minnesota Press, 2014.

British Thoracic Society and Scottish Intercollegiate Guidelines Network. *British Guideline on the Management of Asthma: A National Clinical Guideline.* Edinburgh: Scottish Intercollegiate Guidelines Network, 2016. https://www.brit-thoracic.org.uk.

Brody, Jane E. "A Breathing Technique Offers Help for People with Asthma." *New York Times,* November 2, 2009. http://www.nytimes.com.

Brookes, Tim. *Catching My Breath: An Asthmatic Explores His Illness.* New York: Times Books, 1994.

Brown, Lyn Mikel, and Carol Gilligan. *Meeting at the Crossroads: Women's Psychology and Girls' Development.* Cambridge, Mass.: Harvard University Press, 1992.

Brown, Phil. *Toxic Exposures: Contested Illnesses and the Environmental Health Movement.* New York: Columbia University Press, 2007.

Brown, Phil, Brian Mayer, Stephen Zavestoski, Theo Luebke, Joshua Mandelbaum, and Sabrina McCormick. "The Health Politics of Asthma: Environmental Justice and Collective Illness Experience in the United States." *Social Science & Medicine* 57, no. 3 (2003): 453–64.

Brownlee, Shannon. *Overtreated: Why Too Much Medicine Is Making Us Sicker and Poorer.* New York: Bloomsbury, 2007.

Bruton, Anne, and George T. Lewith. "The Buteyko Breathing Technique for Asthma: A Review." *Complementary Therapies in Medicine* 13, no. 1 (2005): 41–46.

Bruton, Anne, and Mike Thomas. "The Role of Breathing Training in Asthma Management." *Current Opinion in Allergy and Clinical Immunology* 11, no. 1 (2011): 53–57.

Bryant-Stephens, Tyra, Cizely Kurian, and Zhongxue Chen. "Brief Report of a Low-Cost Street-Corner Methodology Used to Assess Inner-City Residents' Awareness and Knowledge about Asthma." *Journal of Urban Health* 88, no. 1 (2011): 156–63.

Bryant-Stephens, Tyra, Shakira Reed-Wells, Maryori Canales, Luzmercy Perez, Marisa Rogers, A. Russell Localio, and Andrea J. Apter. "Home Visits Are Needed to Address Asthma Health Disparities in Adults." *Journal of Allergy and Clinical Immunology* 138, no. 6 (2016): 1526–30.

Burgess, John, Buddhini Ekanayake, Adrian Lowe, David Dunt, Francis Thien, and Shyamali C. Dharmage. "Systematic Review of the Effectiveness of Breathing Retraining in Asthma Management." *Expert Review of Respiratory Medicine* 5, no. 6 (2011): 789–807.

Buteyko, K. P. "Interview with K. P. Buteyko" (1982). In *The Buteyko Method: An Experience of Use in Medicine*. Moscow: Patriot, 1990. http://www.buteyko .ru/eng/interw.shtml.

Callander, Emily J., and Deborah J. Schofield. "Effect of Asthma on Falling into Poverty: The Overlooked Costs of Illness." *Annals of Allergy, Asthma & Immunology* 114, no. 5 (2015): 374–78.

Canguilhem, Georges. *On the Normal and the Pathological*. Berlin: Springer Science & Business Media, 2012.

Celenza, Antonio, Jane Fothergill, Emil Kupek, and Rory J. Shaw. "Thunderstorm Associated Asthma: A Detailed Analysis of Environmental Factors." *BMJ* 312, no. 7031 (1996): 604–7.

Centers for Disease Control and Prevention. "Asthma: Data, Statistics, and Surveillance." Last modified September 8, 2016. https://www.cdc.gov.

———. "National Health Interview Survey (NHIS) Data—2015 Release." Last modified September 2017. https://www.cdc.gov/nchs/nhis/nhis_2015_data_release .htm.

———. "Vital Signs: Asthma in the U.S." Last modified May 2011. https://www .cdc.gov/vitalsigns/asthma/index.html.

Chan, Yu-Feng Yvonne, Pei Wang, Linda Rogers, Nicole L. Tignor, Micol Zweig, Steven G. Hershman, Nicholas Genes, et al. "The Asthma Mobile Health Study, a Large-Scale Clinical Observational Study Using ResearchKit." *Nature Biotechnology* 35, no. 4 (2017): 354–62.

Charmaz, Kathy. *Good Days, Bad Days: The Self in Chronic Illness and Time*. New Brunswick, N.J.: Rutgers University Press, 1991.

Chen, Mel Y. *Animacies: Biopolitics, Racial Mattering, and Queer Affect*. Durham, N.C.: Duke University Press, 2012.

Chen, Nancy N. *Breathing Spaces: Qigong, Psychiatry, and Healing in China*. New York: Columbia University Press, 2003.

Choy, Timothy. *Ecologies of Comparison: An Ethnography of Endangerment in Hong Kong*. Durham, N.C.: Duke University Press, 2011.

Chung, Kian Fan. "New Treatments for Severe Treatment-Resistant Asthma: Targeting the Right Patient." *The Lancet Respiratory Medicine* 1, no. 8 (2013): 639–52.

Chung, Kian Fan, P. Godard, E. Adelroth, J. Ayres, N. Barnes, P. Barnes, E. Bel, et al. "Difficult/Therapy-Resistant Asthma: The Need for an Integrated Approach to Define Clinical Phenotypes, Evaluate Risk Factors, Understand Pathophysiology and Find Novel Therapies." *European Respiratory Journal* 13 (1999): 1198–1208.

Chung, Kian Fan, Sally E. Wenzel, Jan L. Brozek, Andrew Bush, Mario Castro, Peter J. Sterk, Ian M. Adcock, et al. "International ERS/ATS Guidelines on Definition, Evaluation and Treatment of Severe Asthma." *European Respiratory Journal* 43 (2014): 343–73.

Clark, Cindy D. "Asthma Episodes: Stigma, Children, and Hollywood Films." *Medical Anthropology Quarterly* 26, no. 1 (2012): 92–115.

Clarke, Adele E., Laura Mamo, Jennifer Ruth Fosket, Jennifer R. Fishman, and Janet K. Shim, eds. *Biomedicalization: Technoscience, Health, and Illness in the U.S.* Durham, N.C.: Duke University Press, 2010.

Clarke, Adele E., Janet K. Shim, Laura Mamo, Jennifer R. Fosket, and Jennifer R. Fishman. "Biomedicalization: Technoscientific Transformations of Health, Illness, and U.S. Biomedicine." *American Sociological Review* 68, no. 2 (2003): 161–94.

Cohen, Sheldon G. "Asthma among the Famous: A Continuing Series." *Allergy and Asthma Proceedings* (1996–2001).

Comstock, Jonah. "Three Lessons Propeller Learned from a Decade in Digital Health." MobiHealthNews, June 21, 2017. http://www.mobihealthnews.com.

Cooper, S., J. Oborne, S. Newton, V. Harrison, J. Thompson Coon, S. Lewis, and A. Tattersfield. "Effect of Two Breathing Exercises (Buteyko and Pranayama) in Asthma: A Randomised Controlled Trial." *Thorax* 58, no. 8 (2003): 674–79.

Corburn, Jason. *Street Science: Community Knowledge and Environmental Health Justice.* Cambridge, Mass.: MIT Press, 2005.

Cowie, Robert L., Diane P. Conley, Margot F. Underwood, and Patricia G. Reader. "A Randomised Controlled Trial of the Buteyko Technique as an Adjunct to Conventional Management of Asthma." *Respiratory Medicine* 102, no. 5 (2008): 726–32.

Cox-Ganser, Jean M., Ju-Hyeong Park, Jerry Roseman, and Steve Game. "Asthma and Asthma Symptoms in Teachers in 50 Elementary Schools in a Large City." *American Journal of Respiratory and Critical Care Medicine* 195 (2017): A2036.

Cretikos, Michelle A., Rinaldo Bellomo, Ken Hillman, Jack Chen, Simon Finfer, and Arthas Flabouris. "Respiratory Rate: The Neglected Vital Sign." *Medical Journal of Australia* 188, no. 11 (2008): 657–59.

Dabrera, G., V. Murray, J. Emberlin, J. G. Ayres, C. Collier, Y. Clewlow, and P. Sachon. "Thunderstorm Asthma: An Overview of the Evidence Base and Implications for Public Health Advice." *QJM: An International Journal of Medicine* 106, no. 3 (2013): 207–17.

D'Amato, Gennaro, G. Liccardi, and G. Frenguelli. "Thunderstorm-Asthma and Pollen Allergy." *Allergy* 62, no. 1 (2007): 11–16.

Danholt, Peter, and Henriette Langstrup. "Medication as Infrastructure: Decentring Self-Care." *Culture Unbound: Journal of Current Cultural Research* 4, no. 3 (2012): 513–32.

Darveaux, Jared, and William W. Busse. "Biologics in Asthma: The Next Step toward Personalized Treatment." *Journal of Allergy and Clinical Immunology: In Practice* 3, no. 2 (2015): 152–60.

Del Giacco, Stefano R., David Firinu, Leif Bjermer, and Kai-Håkon Carlsen. "Exercise and Asthma: An Overview." *European Clinical Respiratory Journal* 2, no. 1 (2015). doi:10.3402/ecrj.v2.27984.

Denvir, Daniel. "Philly School District Blocks a Federal Study after Health Risks Are Exposed." My City Paper, May 8, 2014. http://mycitypaper.com.

Diamant, Zuzana, J. Diderik Boot, and J. Christian Virchow. "Summing Up 100 Years of Asthma." Respiratory Medicine 101, no. 3 (2007): 378–88.

"Discover the Gadgets That Are Improving Treatments for Asthma." Guardian, April 28, 2017. https://www.theguardian.com.

Downey, Gary Lee, and Teun Zuiderent-Jerak. "Making and Doing: Engagement and Reflexive Learning in STS." In The Handbook of Science and Technology Studies, 4th ed., edited by Ulrike Felt, Rayvon Fouche, Clark A. Miller, and Laurel Smith-Doerr, 223–53. Cambridge, Mass.: MIT Press, 2017.

Dumit, Joseph. Drugs for Life: How Pharmaceutical Companies Define Our Health. Durham, N.C.: Duke University Press, 2012.

Elias, Jack A., Zhou Zhu, Geoffrey Chupp, and Robert J. Homer. "Airway Remodeling in Asthma." Journal of Clinical Investigation 104, no. 8 (1999): 1001–6.

Eng, Quentin Lefebvre, Thomas Vandergoten Eng, Eric Derom, Emilie Marchandise, and Giuseppe Liistro. "Testing Spirometers: Are the Standard Curves of the American Thoracic Society Sufficient?" Respiratory Care 59, no. 12 (2014): 1895–1904.

Englund, Harri. "Ethnography after Globalism: Migration and Emplacement in Malawi." American Ethnologist 29, no. 2 (2002): 261–86.

Epstein, Steven. Impure Science: AIDS, Activism, and the Politics of Knowledge. Berkeley: University of California Press, 1996.

"Excessive Heat, Air Quality 'Code Orange' Warning Issued for Philly and Surrounding Areas." NewsWorks Tonight, WHYY-FM, July 13, 2017. http://www.newsworks.org.

Feyler, Nan. "The Impact of Housing Quality on Children's Health." Lecture, Philadelphia Department of Public Health, Philadelphia, February 2015.

Fitzpatrick, Anne M., W. Gerald Teague, Deborah A. Meyers, Stephen P. Peters, Xingnan Li, Huashi Li, Sally E. Wenzel, et al. "Heterogeneity of Severe Asthma in Childhood: Confirmation by Cluster Analysis of Children in the National Institutes of Health/National Heart, Lung, and Blood Institute Severe Asthma Research Program." Journal of Allergy and Clinical Immunology 127, no. 2 (2011): 382–89.

Fletcher, Christopher M. "Environmental Sensitivity: Equivocal Illness in the Context of Place." Transcultural Psychiatry 43, no. 1 (2006): 86–105.

Fortun, Kim. "Ethnography in Late Industrialism." Cultural Anthropology 27, no. 3 (2012): 446–64.

———. "Ethnography in/of/as Open Systems." Reviews in Anthropology 32, no. 2 (2003): 171–90.

———. "Scaling and Visualizing Multi-sited Ethnography." In Multi-sited Ethnography: Theory, Praxis and Locality in Contemporary Research, edited by Mark-Anthony Falzon, 73–87. New York: Routledge, 2009.

Fortun, Kim, and Michael Fortun. "Anthropologies of the Sciences: Thinking across Strata." In *Exotic No More: Anthropologies on the Front Lines*, 2nd ed., edited by Jeremy MacClancy. Chicago: University of Chicago Press, forthcoming.

Foucault, Michel. *The Birth of the Clinic: An Archaeology of Medical Perception*. Translated by A. M. Sheridan Smith. London: Tavistock, 1973.

———. *Power/Knowledge: Selected Interviews and Other Writings, 1972–1977*. Translated and edited by Colin Gordon. New York: Harvester Wheatsheaf, 1980.

Freifeld, Clark C., Rumi Chunara, Sumiko R. Mekaru, Emily H. Chan, Taha Kass-Hout, Anahi Ayala Iacucci, and John S. Brownstein. "Participatory Epidemiology: Use of Mobile Phones for Community-Based Health Reporting." *PLOS Medicine* 7, no. 12 (2010). doi:10.1371/journal.pmed.1000376.

Frickel, Scott, Sahra Gibbon, Jeff Howard, Joanna Kempner, Gwen Ottinger, and David J. Hess. "Undone Science: Charting Social Movement and Civil Society Challenges to Research Agenda Setting." *Science, Technology, & Human Values* 35, no. 4 (2010): 444–73.

Gabrys, Jennifer. *Program Earth: Environmental Sensing Technology and the Making of a Computational Planet*. Minneapolis: University of Minnesota Press, 2016.

Gerritsen, Jorrit, Gerard H. Koëter, Dirkje S. Postma, Jan P. Schouten, and Klaas Knol. "Prognosis of Asthma from Childhood to Adulthood." *American Review of Respiratory Disease* 140, no. 5 (1989): 1325–30.

Gibson, Mary, ed. *To Breathe Freely: Risk, Consent, and Air*. Totowa, N.J.: Rowman & Allanheld, 1985.

Gilligan, Carol. *In a Different Voice: Psychological Theory and Women's Development*. Cambridge, Mass.: Harvard University Press, 1982.

Girsh, Leonard S., Elliot Shubin, Charles Dick, and Frederic A. Schulaner. "A Study on the Epidemiology of Asthma in Children in Philadelphia: The Relation of Weather and Air Pollution to Peak Incidence of Asthmatic Attacks." *Journal of Allergy and Clinical Immunology* 39, no. 6 (1967): 347–57.

Global Initiative for Asthma. *Global Strategy for Asthma Management and Prevention*. Updated ed. N.p.: GINA, 2018. http://ginasthma.org.

Gold, Diane R., and Rosalind Wright. "Population Disparities in Asthma." *Annual Review of Public Health* 26 (2005): 89–113.

Good, Byron J. *Medicine, Rationality, and Experience: An Anthropological Perspective*. Cambridge: Cambridge University Press, 1994.

Good, Mary-Jo DelVecchio. "The Medical Imaginary and the Biotechnical Embrace: Subjective Experiences of Clinical Scientists and Patients." In *A Reader in Medical Anthropology: Theoretical Trajectories, Emergent Realities*, edited by Byron J. Good, Michael M. J. Fischer, Sarah S. Willen, and Mary-Jo DelVecchio Good, 272–83. Malden, Mass.: Blackwell, 2010.

Górska, Magdalena. *Breathing Matters: Feminist Intersectional Politics of Vulnerability*. Linköping, Sweden: Linköping University, 2016.

Graham, Loren R. *Science in Russia and the Soviet Union: A Short History.* New York: Cambridge University Press, 1993.

Graham, Tess. *Relief from Snoring and Sleep Apnoea: A Step-by-Step Guide to Restful Sleep and Better Health through Changing the Way You Breathe.* Camberwell, Victoria: Penguin Australia, 2012.

Greene, Jeremy A. *Prescribing by Numbers: Drugs and the Definition of Disease.* Baltimore: Johns Hopkins University Press, 2006.

Grosz, Elizabeth. *Time Travels: Feminism, Nature, Power.* Durham, N.C.: Duke University Press, 2005.

Grundstein, Andrew, Stefanie Ebelt Sarnat, Mitchel Klein, Marshall Shepherd, Luke Naeher, Thomas Mote, and Paige Tolbert. "Thunderstorm-Associated Asthma in Atlanta, Georgia." *Thorax* 63, no. 7 (2008): 659–60.

Hahn, Tomie. *Sensational Knowledge: Embodying Culture through Japanese Dance.* Middletown, Conn.: Wesleyan University Press, 2007.

Hamington, Maurice. *Embodied Care: Jane Addams, Maurice Merleau-Ponty, and Feminist Ethics.* Champaign: University of Illinois Press, 2004.

Han, Clara. *Life in Debt: Times of Care and Violence in Neoliberal Chile.* Berkeley: University of California Press, 2012.

Harding, Anne. "Fernando Martinez: Seeking to Solve the Puzzle of Asthma." *The Lancet* 368, no. 9537 (2006): 725.

Hassan, Zahra Mohamed, Nermine Mounir Riad, and Fatma Hassan Ahmed. "Effect of Buteyko Breathing Technique on Patients with Bronchial Asthma." *Egyptian Journal of Chest Diseases and Tuberculosis* 61, no. 4 (2012): 235–41.

Hess, David J. "Medical Modernisation, Scientific Research Fields and the Epistemic Politics of Health Social Movements." *Sociology of Health & Illness* 26, no. 6 (2004): 695–709.

Holgate, Stephen T. "Pathogenesis of Asthma." *Clinical & Experimental Allergy* 38, no. 6 (2008): 872–97.

Howard, John. "NIOSH and Schools." Lecture, National Institute for Occupational Safety and Health, Washington, D.C., November 9, 2015.

Icahn School of Medicine at Mount Sinai. *Asthma Health App, U.S. Participants.* Accessed March 1, 2018. http://apps.icahn.mssm.edu/asthma.

Ingold, Tim. *The Life of Lines.* New York: Routledge, 2015.

Irigaray, Luce. *The Forgetting of Air in Martin Heidegger.* Austin: University of Texas Press, 1999.

Ivanova, Dara, Iris Wallenburg, and Roland Bal. "Care in Place: A Case Study of Assembling a Carescape." *Sociology of Health & Illness* 38, no. 8 (2016): 1336–49.

Jackson, Daniel J., James E. Gern, and Robert F. Lemanske. "The Contributions of Allergic Sensitization and Respiratory Pathogens to Asthma Inception." *Journal of Allergy and Clinical Immunology* 137, no. 3 (2016): 659–65.

Jackson, Mark. "Asthma, Illness, and Identity." *The Lancet* 372, no. 9643 (2008): 1030–31.

———. *Asthma: The Biography*. Oxford: Oxford University Press, 2009.

James, Alan. "Airway Remodeling in Asthma." *Current Opinion in Pulmonary Medicine* 11, no. 1 (2005): 1–6.

Jena, Anupam B., Oliver Ho, Dana P. Goldman, and Pinar Karaca-Mandic. "The Impact of the US Food and Drug Administration Chlorofluorocarbon Ban on Out-of-Pocket Costs and Use of Albuterol Inhalers among Individuals with Asthma." *JAMA Internal Medicine* 175, no. 7 (2015): 1171–79.

Joachim, Gloria, and Sonia Acorn. "Living with Chronic Illness: The Interface of Stigma and Normalization." *Canadian Journal of Nursing Research* 32, no. 3 (2000): 37–48.

Jutel, Annemarie Goldstein. *Putting a Name to It: Diagnosis in Contemporary Society*. Baltimore: Johns Hopkins University Press, 2011.

Keet, Corinne A., Meredith C. McCormack, Craig E. Pollack, Roger D. Peng, Emily McGowan, and Elizabeth C. Matsui. "Neighborhood Poverty, Urban Residence, Race/Ethnicity, and Asthma: Rethinking the Inner-City Asthma Epidemic." *Journal of Allergy and Clinical Immunology* 135, no. 3 (2015): 655–62.

Keirns, Carla C. "Better Than Nature: The Changing Treatment of Asthma and Hay Fever in the United States, 1910–1945." *Studies in History and Philosophy of Science Part C* 34, no. 3 (2003): 511–31.

Kenner, Alison. "Asthma on the Move: How Mobile Apps Remediate Risk for Disease Management." *Health, Risk & Society* 17, nos. 7–8 (2016): 510–29.

———. "The Healthy Asthmatic." *M/C Journal* 16, no. 6 (2013).

Kittay, Eva Feder. *Love's Labor: Essays on Women, Equality, and Dependency*. New York: Routledge, 1999.

———. "Taking Dependency Seriously: The Family and Medical Leave Act Considered in Light of the Social Organization of Dependency Work and Gender Equality." *Hypatia* 10, no. 1 (1995): 8–29.

Klawiter, Maren. *The Biopolitics of Breast Cancer: Changing Cultures of Disease and Activism*. Minneapolis: University of Minnesota Press, 2008.

Knowles, Scott Gabriel. "Learning from Disaster? The History of Technology and the Future of Disaster Research." *Technology and Culture* 55, no. 4 (2014): 773–84.

Krieger, James K., Tim K. Takaro, Carol Allen, Lin Song, Marcia Weaver, Sanders Chai, and Phillip Dickey. "The Seattle–King County Healthy Homes Project: Implementation of a Comprehensive Approach to Improving Indoor Environmental Quality for Low-Income Children with Asthma." Supplement, *Environmental Health Perspectives* 110, no. 2 (2002): 311.

Kroll-Smith, Steve, Philip M. Brown, and Valerie Jan Gunter, eds. *Illness and the Environment: A Reader in Contested Medicine*. New York: New York University Press, 2000.

Kruse, Julie. *Lead Hazard Control and Healthy Homes*. Washington, D.C.: U.S. Department of Housing and Urban Development, 2016. http://nlihc.org.

Lane, Taylor S., Julie Armin, and Judith S. Gordon. "Online Recruitment Methods for Web-Based and Mobile Health Studies: A Review of the Literature." *Journal of Medical Internet Research* 17, no. 7 (2015). doi:10.2196/jmir.4359.

Lang, David M., and Marcia Polansky. "Patterns of Asthma Mortality in Philadelphia from 1969 to 1991." *New England Journal of Medicine* 331 (1994): 1542–46.

Langstrup, Henriette. "Chronic Care Infrastructures and the Home." *Sociology of Health & Illness* 35, no. 7 (2013): 1008–22.

Latour, Bruno. "How to Talk about the Body? The Normative Dimension of Science Studies." *Body & Society* 10, nos. 2–3 (2004): 205–29.

Lefebvre, Henri. *Rhythmanalysis: Space, Time and Everyday Life*. Translated by Stuart Elden and Gerald Moore. New York: Continuum, 2004.

Lockey, Richard F. "Defining Phenotypes: Expanding Our Understanding of Asthma Challenges in Treating a Heterogeneous Disease." PowerPoint presentation, Division of Allergy and Immunology, Department of Internal Medicine, University of South Florida College of Medicine, 2009. http://www.worldallergy.org.

Loh, Penn, and Jodi Sugerman-Brozan. "Environmental Justice Organizing for Environmental Health: Case Study on Asthma and Diesel Exhaust in Roxbury, Massachusetts." *Annals of the American Academy of Political and Social Science* 584, no. 1 (2002): 110–24.

Lötvall, Jan, Cezmi A. Akdis, Leonard B. Bacharier, Leif Bjermer, Thomas B. Casale, Adnan Custovic, Robert F. Lemanske, Andrew J. Wardlaw, Sally E. Wenzel, and Paul A. Greenberger. "Asthma Endotypes: A New Approach to Classification of Disease Entities within the Asthma Syndrome." *Journal of Allergy and Clinical Immunology* 127, no. 2 (2011): 355–60.

Maantay, Juliana. "Asthma and Air Pollution in the Bronx: Methodological and Data Considerations in Using GIS for Environmental Justice and Health Research." *Health & Place* 13, no. 1 (2007): 32–56.

Malfitano, Nicholas. "Philadelphia Dismissed from Lawsuit over Death of 12-Year-Old Who Didn't Receive Asthma Meds at School." Pennsylvania Record, May 14, 2015. http://pennrecord.com.

Marcus, George E. "Ethnography in/of the World System: The Emergence of Multi-sited Ethnography." *Annual Review of Anthropology* 24 (1995): 95–117.

Martin, A. J., L. I. Landau, and P. D. Phelan. "Asthma from Childhood at Age 21: The Patient and His Disease." *British Medical Journal (Clinical Research Edition)* 284, no. 6313 (1982): 380–82.

Martin, Aryn, Natasha Myers, and Ana Viseu. "The Politics of Care in Technoscience." *Social Studies of Science* 45, no. 5 (2015): 625–41.

Massey, Doreen. *For Space*. London: Sage, 2005.

Maynard, Ronald J. "Controlling Death—Compromising Life: Chronic Disease, Prognostication, and the New Biotechnologies." *Medical Anthropology Quarterly* 20, no. 2 (2006): 212–34.

McHugh, Patrick, Fergus Aitcheson, Bruce Duncan, and Frank Houghton. "Buteyko Breathing Technique for Asthma: An Effective Intervention." *New Zealand Medical Journal (Online)* 116, no. 1187 (2003).

McKeown, Patrick. *Close Your Mouth: Buteyko Breathing Clinic Self Help Manual—Stop Asthma, Hay Fever and Nasal Congestion Permanently.* Galway: Buteyko Books, 2004.

———. *The Oxygen Advantage: The Simple, Scientifically Proven Breathing Techniques for a Healthier, Slimmer, Faster, and Fitter You.* New York: William Morrow, 2015.

McLean, Diane E., Shawn Bowen, Karen Drezner, Amy Rowe, Peter Sherman, Scott Schroeder, Karen Redlener, and Irwin Redlener. "Asthma among Homeless Children: Undercounting and Undertreating the Underserved." *Archives of Pediatrics & Adolescent Medicine* 158, no. 3 (2004): 244–49.

Melgert, Barbro N., Anuradha Ray, Machteld N. Hylkema, Wim Timens, and Dirkje S. Postma. "Are There Reasons Why Adult Asthma Is More Common in Females?" *Current Allergy and Asthma Reports* 7, no. 2 (2007): 143–50.

Meyer, John M. *Engaging the Everyday: Environmental Social Criticism and the Resonance Dilemma.* Cambridge, Mass.: MIT Press, 2015.

Milligan, Ki Lee, Elizabeth Matsui, and Hemant Sharma. "Asthma in Urban Children: Epidemiology, Environmental Risk Factors, and the Public Health Domain." *Current Allergy and Asthma Report* 16, no. 4 (2016). doi:10.1007/s11882-016-0609-6.

Mitman, Gregg. *Breathing Space: How Allergies Shape Our Lives and Landscapes.* New Haven, Conn.: Yale University Press, 2007.

Mol, Annemarie. *The Logic of Care: Health and the Problem of Patient Choice.* London: Routledge, 2008.

Mol, Annemarie, Ingunn Moser, and Jeannette Pols, eds. *Care in Practice: On Tinkering in Clinics, Homes and Farms.* Bielefeld, Germany: Transcript-Verlag, 2010.

Moore, Wendy C., Deborah A. Meyers, Sally E. Wenzel, W. Gerald Teague, Huashi Li, Xingnan Li, Ralph D'Agostino Jr., et al. "Identification of Asthma Phenotypes Using Cluster Analysis in the Severe Asthma Research Program." *American Journal of Respiratory and Critical Care Medicine* 181, no. 4 (2010): 315–23.

Moorman, Jeanne E., Lara J. Akinbami, C. M. Bailey, H. S. Zahran, M. E. King, C. A. Johnson, and X. Liu. "National Surveillance of Asthma: United States, 2001–2010." *Vital & Health Statistics, Series 3, Analytical and Epidemiological Studies* 35 (2012): 1–58.

Munn, Nancy D. "The Cultural Anthropology of Time: A Critical Essay." *Annual Review of Anthropology* 21, no. 1 (1992): 93–123.

Murphy, Michelle. *Seizing the Means of Reproduction: Entanglements of Feminism, Health, and Technoscience.* Durham, N.C.: Duke University Press, 2012.

———. *Sick Building Syndrome and the Problem of Uncertainty: Environmental Politics, Technoscience, and Women Workers.* Durham, N.C.: Duke University Press, 2006.

———. "Unsettling Care: Troubling Transnational Itineraries of Care in Feminist Health Practices." *Social Studies of Science* 45, no. 5 (2015): 717–37.

Nading, Alex M. *Mosquito Trails: Ecology, Health, and the Politics of Entanglement.* Berkeley: University of California Press, 2014.

Natanson, Elad. "Digital Therapeutics: The Future of Health Care Will be App-Based." *Forbes,* July 24, 2017. https://www.forbes.com.

National Asthma Education and Prevention Program. *Expert Panel Report 3: Guidelines for the Diagnosis and Management of Asthma—Summary Report 2007.* NIH Publication 08-5846. Bethesda, Md.: National Heart, Lung, and Blood Institute, National Institutes of Health, October 2007. https://www.nhlbi.nih.gov.

National Heart, Lung, and Blood Institute. *Putting the Guidelines Implementation Panel Report in Motion: A Plan of Action for the National Asthma Control Initiative.* NIH Publication 10-7543. Bethesda, Md.: National Heart, Lung, and Blood Institute, National Institutes of Health, April 2010. https://www.nhlbi.nih.gov.

Nixon, Rob. *Slow Violence and the Environmentalism of the Poor.* Cambridge, Mass.: Harvard University Press, 2011.

Novozhilov, Andrey. *Living without Asthma: The Buteyko Method.* 2nd ed. Friedberg, Germany: Mobiwell Verlag, 2004.

Nurmagambetov, Tursynbek, Robin Kuwahara, and Paul Garbe. "The Economic Burden of Asthma in the United States, 2008–2013." *Annals of the American Thoracic Society* 15, no. 3 (2018): 348–56.

O'Connor, Elizabeth, Carrie D. Patnode, Brittany U. Burda, David I. Buckley, and Evelyn P. Whitlock. *Breathing Exercises and/or Retraining Techniques in the Treatment of Asthma: Comparative Effectiveness.* AHRQ Publication 12-EHC092-EF. Rockville, Md.: Agency for Healthcare Research and Quality, 2012. https://www.ncbi.nlm.nih.gov/books/NBK109355.

Opat, A. J., M. M. Cohen, M. J. Bailey, and M. J. Abramson. "A Clinical Trial of the Buteyko Breathing Technique in Asthma as Taught by a Video." *Journal of Asthma* 37, no. 7 (2000): 557–64.

Orso, Anna. "Why You're Seeing More Homelessness in Center City, and How Philly Is Responding." Billy Penn, May 16, 2016. https://billypenn.com.

Pennsylvania Department of Health. *2015 Asthma Prevalence Report.* Harrisburg: Pennsylvania Department of Health, 2015. http://www.health.pa.gov.

Philadelphia Department of Public Health. *Community Health Assessment.* Philadelphia: Department of Public Health, 2014. http://www.phila.gov.

"Philadelphia's Dirty Schools May Be Making Students and Teachers Sick." Video, *America Tonight,* Aljazeera America, November 30, 2015. http://america.aljazeera.com/watch/shows/america-tonight.html.

Pink, Sarah. "From Embodiment to Emplacement: Re-thinking Competing Bodies, Senses and Spatialities." *Sport, Education and Society* 16, no. 3 (2011): 343–55.

"A Plea to Abandon Asthma as a Disease Concept." *The Lancet* 368, no. 9537 (2006): 705.

Pols, Jeannette. *Care at a Distance: On the Closeness of Technology.* Chicago: University of Chicago Press, 2012.

———. "Knowing Patients: Turning Patient Knowledge into Science." *Science, Technology, & Human Values* 39, no. 1 (2013): 73–97.

Prasanna, K. B., K. R. Sowmiya, and C. M. Dhileeban. "Effect of Buteyko Breathing Exercise in Newly Diagnosed Asthmatic Patients." *International Journal of Medicine and Public Health* 5, no. 1 (2015): 77–81.

Prem, Venkatesan, Ramesh Chandra Sahoo, and Prabha Adhikari. "Comparison of the Effects of Buteyko and Pranayama Breathing Techniques on Quality of Life in Patients with Asthma: A Randomized Controlled Trial." *Clinical Rehabilitation* 27, no. 2 (2013): 133–41.

Propeller Health. "Asthmapolis Relaunches as Propeller Health to Advance Broader Respiratory Mission." Press release, September 10, 2013. https://www.propellerhealth.com/2013/09/10.

———. *Live Your Life without Limits.* Video, 2016. https://vimeo.com/156787142.

———. "Louisville Data Findings to Aid City Leaders in Reducing Burden of Asthma." Press release, June 28, 2017. https://www.propellerhealth.com/2017/06/28.

———. "Propeller Health Receives FDA Clearance for the Propeller Platform in Association with GSK's Ellipta Inhaler." Press release, November 7, 2016. https://www.propellerhealth.com/2016/11/07.

———. *What Is Propeller?* Video, 2010. https://vimeo.com/12175855.

Public Health Institute. "PHI's Center for Climate Change and Health Announces Learning Collaborative for Urban Health Departments." October 27, 2015. http://www.phi.org/news-events.

Puig de la Bellacasa, María. "Making Time for Soil: Technoscientific Futurity and the Pace of Care." *Social Studies of Science* 45, no. 5 (2015): 691–716.

———. "Matters of Care in Technoscience: Assembling Neglected Things." *Social Studies of Science* 41, no. 1 (2011): 85–106.

———. *Matters of Care: Speculative Ethics in More Than Human Worlds.* Minneapolis: University of Minnesota Press, 2017.

Rackemann, Francis M. "Intrinsic Asthma." *Journal of Allergy and Clinical Immunology* 11, no. 2 (1940): 147–62.

———. "A Working Classification of Asthma." *American Journal of Medicine* 3, no. 5 (1947): 601–6.

Ram, Felix S. F., E. A. Holloway, and P. W. Jones. "Breathing Retraining for Asthma." *Respiratory Medicine* 97, no. 5 (2003): 501–7.

"Ranking Member Cummings and Chairman Sanders Investigate Staggering Price Increases for Generic Drugs." Bernie Sanders, U.S. Senator for Vermont, website, October 2014. https://www.sanders.senate.gov.

Rao, Carol Y., Margaret A. Riggs, Ginger L. Chew, Michael L. Muilenberg, Peter S. Thorne, David Van Sickle, Kevin H. Dunn, and Clive Brown. "Characterization of Airborne Molds, Endotoxins, and Glucans in Homes in New Orleans after Hurricanes Katrina and Rita." *Applied and Environmental Microbiology* 73, no. 5 (2007): 1630–34.

Reddel, Helen K., D. Robin Taylor, Eric D. Bateman, Louis-Philippe Boulet, Homer A. Boushey, William W. Busse, Thomas B. Casale, et al. "An Official American Thoracic Society/European Respiratory Society Statement: Asthma Control and Exacerbations—Standardizing Endpoints for Clinical Asthma Trials and Clinical Practice." *American Journal of Respiratory and Critical Care Medicine* 180, no. 1 (2009): 59–99.

Reno, Joshua. "Beyond Risk: Emplacement and the Production of Environmental Evidence." *American Ethnologist* 38, no. 3 (2011): 516–30.

Romero, Melissa. "Mapping the 29 High-Rises under Construction in Philly Right Now." Curbed Philadelphia, January 23, 2018. https://philly.curbed.com.

Rona, Roberto J. "Asthma and Poverty." *Thorax* 55, no. 3 (2000): 239–44.

Roseman, Jerry. "Can We Make Philadelphia Schools Safer, Healthier?" Healthy Kids (blog), *Philadelphia Inquirer,* April 6, 2016. http://www.philly.com.

———. "A Matter of Health and Safety." *American Educator* 40, no. 4 (2017): 34–39.

Rosenthal, Elizabeth. "The Soaring Cost of a Simple Breath." *New York Times,* October 12, 2013. http://www.nytimes.com.

Ruckenstein, Minna, and Natasha Dow Schüll. "The Datafication of Health." *Annual Review of Anthropology* 46 (2017): 261–78.

Sanz, Camilo. "Out-of-Sync Cancer Care: Health Insurance Companies, Biomedical Practices, and Clinical Time in Colombia." *Medical Anthropology* 26, no. 3 (2017): 187–201.

Schmidt, Charles W. "Pollen Overload: Seasonal Allergies in a Changing Climate." *Environmental Health Perspectives* 124, no. 4 (2016): A70–75.

School District of Philadelphia. *Use of Medications/Medical Technology.* August 24, 2011. https://www.philasd.org.

Schüll, Natasha Dow. "Data for Life: Wearable Technology and the Design of Self-Care." *BioSocieties* 11, no. 3 (2016): 317–33.

Shapiro, Nicholas. "Attuning to the Chemosphere: Domestic Formaldehyde, Bodily Reasoning, and the Chemical Sublime." *Cultural Anthropology* 30, no. 3 (2015): 368–93.

Siroux, Valérie, Anne Boudier, Jean Bousquet, Jean-Louis Bresson, Jean-Luc Cracowski, Joane Ferran, Frédéric Gormand, et al. "Phenotypic Determinants of Uncontrolled Asthma." *Journal of Allergy and Clinical Immunology* 124, no. 4 (2009): 681–87.

Sloterdijk, Peter. *Bubbles: Spheres I.* Cambridge: MIT Press, 2011.

———. *Terror from the Air.* Cambridge: MIT Press, 2009.

Smith, Susan Lampert. "Researcher Uses GPS to Find Asthma Causes." University of Wisconsin–Madison News, April 2, 2009. https://news.wisc.edu.

Stark, Jennifer, and Russell Stark. *The Buteyko Method and the Carbon Dioxide Syndrome.* Coorparoo, Queensland: Buteyko Works, 2002.

Stein, Renato T., and Fernando D. Martinez. "Asthma Phenotypes in Childhood: Lessons from an Epidemiological Approach." *Paediatric Respiratory Reviews* 5, no. 2 (2004): 155–61.

Stevenson, Lisa. *Life beside Itself: Imagining Care in the Canadian Arctic.* Berkeley: University of California Press, 2014.

Stewart, Kathleen. "Atmospheric Attunements." *Environment and Planning D: Society and Space* 29, no. 3 (2011): 445–53.

Strathern, Marilyn. *Partial Connections.* Walnut Creek, Calif.: AltaMira Press, 2005.

Strauss, Valeria. "Girl Dies after Getting Sick at School without Nurse." *Washington Post,* October 12, 2013. https://www.washingtonpost.com.

Su, Jason G., Meredith A. Barrett, Kelly Henderson, Olivier Humblet, Ted Smith, James W. Sublett, LaQuandra Nesbitt, et al. "Feasibility of Deploying Inhaler Sensors to Identify the Impacts of Environmental Triggers and Built Environment Factors on Asthma Short-Acting Bronchodilator Use." *Environmental Health Perspectives* 125, no. 2 (2017): 254–61.

Thrift, Nigel. *Non-representational Theory: Space, Politics, Affect.* New York: Routledge, 2008.

Ticktin, Miriam I. *Casualties of Care: Immigration and the Politics of Humanitarianism in France.* Berkeley: University of California Press, 2011.

Trnka, Susanna. *One Blue Child: Asthma, Responsibility, and the Politics of Global Health.* Stanford, Calif.: Stanford University Press, 2017.

Tronto, Joan C. "Beyond Gender Difference to a Theory of Care." *Signs: Journal of Women in Culture and Society* 12, no. 4 (1987): 644–63.

———. *Moral Boundaries: A Political Argument for an Ethic of Care.* New York: Routledge, 1993.

U.S. Global Change Research Program. *The Impacts of Climate Change on Human Health in the United States: A Scientific Assessment.* Washington, D.C.: USGCRP, 2016. https://health2016.globalchange.gov.

van Dijck, José, and Thomas Poell. "Understanding the Promises and Premises of Online Health Platforms." *Big Data & Society* 3, no. 1 (2016). doi:10.1177/2053951716654173.

Van Leuvan, Chris H., and Imogen Mitchell. "Missed Opportunities? An Observational Study of Vital Sign Measurements." *Critical Care and Resuscitation* 10, no. 2 (2008): 111–15.

Van Sickle, David. "Diagnosis and Management of Asthma in the Medical Marketplace of India: Implications for Efforts to Improve Global Respiratory Health." In *Anthropology and Public Health: Bridging Differences in Culture and Society,* 2nd ed., edited by Robert A. Hahn and Marcia C. Inhorn, 65–93. New York: Oxford University Press, 2009.

Van Sickle, David, and Anne L. Wright, "Navajo Perceptions of Asthma and Asthma Medications: Clinical Implications." *Pediatrics* 108, no. 1 (2001). doi:10.1542/peds.108.1.e11.

von Mutius, Erika, and Fernando D. Martinez. "Inconclusive Results of Randomized Trials of Prenatal Vitamin D for Asthma Prevention in Offspring: Curbing the Enthusiasm." *JAMA* 315, no. 4 (2016): 347–48.

Vuckovic, Nancy. "Fast Relief: Buying Time with Medications." *Medical Anthropology Quarterly* 13, no. 1 (1999): 51–68.

Wallis, Daniel N., Julian Webb, Duncan Brooke, Beata Brookes, Ruth Brown, Alice Findlay, Miriam Harris, et al. "A Major Outbreak of Asthma Associated with a Thunderstorm: Experience of Accident and Emergency Departments and Patients' Characteristics." *BMJ* 312, no. 7031 (1996): 601–4.

Wener, Reinier R. L., and Elisabeth H. Bel. "Severe Refractory Asthma: An Update." *European Respiratory Review* 22 (2013): 227–35.

Wenzel, Sally E. "Asthma Phenotypes: The Evolution from Clinical to Molecular Approaches." *Nature Medicine* 18, no. 5 (2012): 716–25.

Whipp, Richard, Barbara Adam, and Ida Sabelis, eds. *Making Time: Time and Management in Modern Organizations.* Oxford: Oxford University Press, 2002.

Whitmarsh, Ian. *Biomedical Ambiguity: Race, Asthma, and the Contested Meaning of Genetic Research in the Caribbean.* Ithaca, N.Y.: Cornell University Press, 2011.

———. "Biomedical Ambivalence: Asthma Diagnosis, the Pharmaceutical, and Other Contradictions in Barbados." *American Ethnologist* 35, no. 1 (2008): 49–63.

Wind, Steven, David Van Sickle, and Anne L. Wright. "Health, Place and Childhood Asthma in Southwest Alaska." *Social Science & Medicine* 58, no. 1 (2004): 75–88.

Windle, Greg. "District Scrambling to Remove Mold at Muñoz-Marin in Time to Open School." *Philadelphia Public Schools Notebook,* August 25, 2017. http://thenotebook.org.

Wolf-Meyer, Matthew. "Therapy, Remedy, Cure: Disorder and the Spatiotemporality of Medicine and Everyday Life." *Medical Anthropology* 33, no. 2 (2014): 144–59.

Wood, Stephanie. "Thunderstorm Asthma: The Night a Deadly Storm took Melbourne's Breath Away." *Sydney Morning Herald,* March 10, 2017. https://www.smh.com.au.

Zhao, Jing, Becky Freeman, and Mu Li. "Can Mobile Phone Apps Influence People's Health Behavior Change? An Evidence Review." *Journal of Medical Internet Research* 18, no. 11 (2016). doi:10.2196/jmir.5692.

acupuncture, 88, 96
Adam, Barbara, 18
aeroallergen concentrations, 4, 163
Affordable Care Act (ACA), 135
AHA. *See* Asthma Health Application
air conditioners, heat islands and, 167
airflow limitations, 37, 38, 44, 45, 46, 61, 197n32
AirNow, 169
air pollution, 3, 19, 143, 145, 148, 152, 153, 160, 166, 206n17; asthma and, 116; grass pollen and, 4; outdoor, 167; pre-exposure to, 163; reducing, 185
air quality, 3, 6, 26, 57, 143, 160, 163, 165; analyzing, 140; differences in, 51; improving, 177; information, 178–79; poor, 79, 81, 150, 170; symptoms and, 51
Air Quality Index (AQI), 146, 152–53, 205n12, 207n30
airway inflammation, 37, 62, 68, 93
albuterol, 1, 2, 30, 32, 42, 73, 131, 133, 193n41
Allen, Dave, 147
allergenicity, 162, 163
allergens, 6, 37, 44, 162, 163
allergic asthma, 2, 11, 38, 54, 58, 75, 131, 197n25, 198n41; definitions

of, 31–32; development of, 65, 80, 98; pathophysiological definitions for, 41; severe, 85, 111
allergies, 11, 81, 85, 92, 127, 163; asthma and, 31–32, 41, 138, 151; food, 133; history of, 42; seasonal, 5, 31, 32, 36, 49; uncontrolled, 86; waxing/waning, 49
Allergy and Asthma Foundation of America, 194n67, 198n1
Allergy and Asthma Network, 127, 129
Allergy and Asthma Proceedings (Cohen), 195n3
allergy shots, 49, 111
American Lung Association, 194n67
American Thoracic Society (ATS), 44, 62, 63, 68, 70, 198n5
Anderson, Gary P., 11, 192n27
antibiotics, 31, 42
apps, 19, 131, 134, 143; breathing technique, 118; development of, 123, 136; disease management, 26, 135; environmental, 142; health, 25, 134; mobile phone, 118, 119; mPower, 136; Propeller, 26, 115, 141, 146; research, 137. *See also* asthma care apps
AQI. *See* Air Quality Index

assessments, 14, 67, 70, 126, 129; clinical, 84, 134; risk, 60–61, 68

asthma: addressing, 10, 62, 182; atopic, 32; characteristics of, 44, 180; childhood, 12, 149; complexity/heterogeneity of, 10–11, 38, 39; developing, 10, 12, 41, 66, 87; dormant, 51, 52; episodic, 10, 11, 30, 34, 48, 57, 66, 72; experiences of, 28, 34, 40–43, 49–50, 53, 54, 75–76, 77; history of, 32, 43, 45, 54, 202n34; intimate/public valences of, 5; late-onset, 38; managing, 3, 10, 13, 14, 113, 145, 146; mild, 10, 23, 48, 50, 52; moderate, 50, 73; non-allergic, 38; occupational, 10; outgrowing, 11, 48–56; rates of, 12, 173–74; real, 29–30, 55; risks for, 63, 64, 117; severe, 23, 24, 31, 36, 50, 63, 69, 111; thunderstorm, 4, 5, 163, 164, 206n23; types of, 30, 35, 36, 40, 54, 58; uncontrolled, 31, 63, 86, 126–27; understanding, 122

asthma action plans, 15, 120, 129, 131, 132, 134, 135, 183

Asthma Ally, 127, 129, 130, 142, 204n15

Asthma and Allergy Foundation of America, 152, 191n3

Asthma App, 139

asthma attacks, 1, 2–3, 24, 29; daytime/nighttime, 7, 61; geocoding, 25; risk of, 67; structural conditions for, 3–4; talking through, 75–76; variations in, 35, 122

asthma care apps, 26, 115, 118, 119, 120, 122, 124, 134, 135, 142, 144, 146, 147, 148, 149; benefits of, 139; designing, 125–27, 129–31, 203n14; science of, 136–41

Asthma Check, 126–27, 129–30

Asthma Edge, 120, 121, 122, 130, 141

asthma epidemic, 4, 6, 12, 19, 20, 27, 117, 119, 156, 161, 166, 184, 192n11, 195n77; attention for, 23, 158; climate change and, 5, 8, 162, 175, 176; data from, 146; emergence of, 63; local, 22; public cost of, 64; as public health issue, 149, 150

Asthma Health Application (AHA), 130, 137, 141, 142, 146, 148, 182; environmental data and, 140; satisfaction with, 138; structure/clarity of, 139

Asthma Health Map, 138

AsthmaMD, 129, 130

Asthma Plan, 140

Asthmapolis, 25, 26, 116, 117

Asthma Readiness and Resilience Project, 165

Asthma Storylines, 127, 128 (fig.), 129

asthma sufferers, 6, 7, 12, 15, 17, 25, 37, 47, 48, 59, 60, 63, 76, 79, 87, 88; BBT and, 112; biographies of, 110–11, 202n34; classification systems by, 32; interviews with, 18, 24, 99, 180, 185; tactics of, 66, 180, 181

atmosphere, 3, 17, 162, 182, 191n4

atmospheric pressure, 143

ATS. See American Thoracic Society

attunement, 18, 34, 66, 72, 73, 79, 81, 89, 99, 164, 178, 180, 181; asthmatic, 35, 41, 57, 65; concept of, 16–17; emplacement and, 60; power of, 83

avoidance measures, 15, 17, 33, 81, 82, 83

awareness, 7, 34, 36, 63, 86, 96, 99, 102, 134, 139, 147, 152; somatic, 29–30, 50; symptom, 57

Baglia, Carol, 105

Bauman, Chris, 105

BBEA. *See* Buteyko Breathing Educators Association

BBEs. *See* Buteyko breathing educators

BBT. *See* Buteyko breathing technique

"Be Air Aware" workshop, 166–67, 171

beta-adrenergic agonist, 202n39

biochemistry, 58, 60, 88, 179

biological differences: population-based research on, 13; scales of, 7

biomedicalization, 7, 8, 16, 19, 25, 28, 48, 55, 56, 87, 89, 93, 161, 184; characteristics of, 26

blood lead levels, 170

Blue Cross, 132, 135, 136

Bowlby, Sophie, 157–58, 192n17

Braun, Lundy, 197n32

breath: counting on, 99–103; playing with/out, 71–79; shortness of, 30, 37, 65

breath control, 75, 77, 78, 184–85; forms of, 180; learning, 83; practicing, 149, 164, 181; techniques for, 17, 180, 181

breathers, 17, 80–81, 82, 149; term, 5–6, 191n5

breath holds, 95, 98–99, 100, 101, 102, 107, 113

breathing, 18, 90, 127, 132, 160, 161, 178; atmosphere and, 17; cycles, 77, 85; deep, 92; difficulties with, 35, 42, 48, 73, 80, 172; focusing on, 74; functional, 56; habitual, 99; inhalers and, 109–13; listening to, 1; normal, 73, 93, 100, 101, 133; pace of, 4; rates of, 90; relaxation and, 94–99; rhythmic, 32, 88, 103; shallow, 69; tracking, 89; voluntary/involuntary, 180, 194n55. *See also* disordered breathing

breathing exercises, 15, 76, 85, 95–96, 98–99, 113, 149; qigong, 199n31; tactile, 86; tracking, 101

breathing space, 3, 177

breathing techniques, 2, 25, 77–78, 93, 97, 106, 180, 200n10, 200n15; developing, 83; disordered breathing and, 77; experimenting with, 73; learning, 99; recommending, 89; rhythms of, 98; using, 75, 76, 78

breathlessness, 2, 4, 11, 30, 35, 61, 111

Breathmobile, 184, 194n67, 199n38; photo of, 184

Brody, Jane, 110, 202n34

bronchitis, 31, 42, 71, 168

bronchodilators, 1, 13, 30, 45, 70, 111, 198n18

Brookes, Tim, 36, 37, 39–40, 56, 67; asthma and, 33–34; on chronic illness, 55

Bryant-Stephens, Tyra, 173–74, 175

Buteyko, Konstantin, 22, 89, 96, 99, 201n31; biographical information on, 201n18; McKeown and, 105; research by, 91–92, 94; teaching by, 106; theory of, 90, 92, 93, 109

Buteyko, Ludmilla, 105

Buteyko breathing educators (BBEs), 25, 85–86, 96–97, 100, 102, 108, 112, 113, 149, 184; archives by, 105; health and, 99; information sharing by, 103, 105, 109; logbooks and, 101; tools of, 95 (fig.); websites of, 89

Buteyko Breathing Educators Association (BBEA), 24–25, 103, 105, 109, 112, 202n32; training standards of, 106

Buteyko breathing technique (BBT), 28, 87, 88, 93, 95, 99, 101, 113, 118, 149, 180, 184; availability of, 112, 181; books on, 201n21; commitment to, 109; described, 24–25; development of, 89–90, 96; impact of, 97, 107, 110; literature on, 92, 201n20; stress and, 96; symptoms and, 181; teaching, 103, 105, 106, 107–8, 107 (fig.), 109; timescales and, 94; using, 88, 96–97, 98, 100, 102, 103, 109

Buteyko Institute of Breathing and Health, 105

Byrne-Ralfs, Christine, 104

Canguilhem, Georges: on respiratory rhythm, 57

carbon dioxide, 92, 93, 162

carbon monoxide, 168, 170

cardiovascular disease, 15

care, 6, 35, 40, 56, 113, 119, 135, 139, 142, 185, 192n17, 199n38, 206n19; as analytic framework, 16; chronic, 23, 118–19; clinical, 61, 94, 181; components of, 7, 46, 120; context-specific, 20; costs of, 15; effective, 183; focus on, 22; implementing, 82–83; iterations of, 15–20; making time for, 89, 103, 105–9; mode of, 16, 17, 149, 194n69, 200n10; pillars of, 79, 82; regimens and, 126; revolutionizing, 118, 136; rhythmic, 88, 106, 181; studying, 131–32; tracing, 16, 21–28, 119–25; webs of, 8, 179

Care Cam app, 131, 134, 135, 136

carescapes, 8, 16, 19, 150, 158, 165, 166, 171, 176, 179; development of, 183; effective, 182; minimal, 178; public health, 20

Catching My Breath: An Asthmatic Explores His Illness (Brookes), 33–34, 40

Caum, Jessica, 165–66

Center City, 151, 160, 161

Centers for Disease Control and Prevention (CDC), 11, 12, 117, 164, 165; asthma action plans and, 120;

asthma care costs and, 15; asthma surveillance data from, 137

Chapman, Saleem, 167; photo of, 171

chemicals, 3, 6, 8, 81, 89, 167, 185

Chen, Nancy, 199n31

chest tightness, 2, 35, 61, 66

Children's Hospital of Philadelphia, 172–73

chlorofluorocarbons (CFCs), ban on, 13

Choy, Tim, 5–6, 191n5, 193n52

chronic conditions, 32, 92, 129, 181–82

Chung, Kian Fan, 202n39

Clarke, Adele, 203n43

classification system, 34, 36, 44, 196n5

Clean Air Act, 153, 205n17

Clean Air Council, 152, 154, 155, 167, 170, 171

Climate and Health Program, 164, 206n24

Climate and Urban Systems Partnership (CUSP), 155, 157, 166, 172, 205n13

climate change, 21, 53, 150, 151–58, 167, 170, 179, 182; asthma epidemic and, 5, 6, 8, 162, 175, 176; dynamics of, 166; environment and, 172; impacts of, 5, 151, 162, 165, 171, 175, 185; planning for, 164; pollen and, 163; public/home environments and, 156; slow violence of, 176; thunderstorm asthma and, 206n23; working knowledge of, 160

Climate, Health, and Home project, 27, 150, 151, 152, 154–59, 166–67, 169, 170, 182, 183

Climate-Ready States and Cities Initiative, 164

clinical protocols, 43, 56, 63

clinical trials, 11, 64, 138

cockroaches, 8
"Code Orange Air Quality Action Day," 152
Code Orange days, 152, 153
Code Red services, 157
cold air, 8, 162
Community Asthma Prevention Program, 173
Community Health Assessment (PDPH), 150
comorbidities, 22, 50, 62
control, 3, 5, 18, 36, 44, 53, 87, 115, 132, 140, 141, 143; achieving, 20; assessing, 67, 70, 126, 129; comfort/companionship and, 81; disease, 64–79; environmental, 10, 17–18, 24, 68, 79–84, 88; future risk in, 60–64; handling, 24, 63, 170, 178; layers of, 78; logic of, 136; monitoring and, 129; preemptive, 73; social, 78–79; tactics for, 67; term, 18, 67
control pause, 100, 101, 102
cooling centers, 152, 153
COPD, 116, 145
Corse, Teija, 153
corticosteroids, 13, 24, 58, 111, 202n39
coughing, 2, 4, 16, 31, 48, 71
CUSP. See Climate and Urban Systems Partnership

dander, 6, 8, 36, 88, 162
data, 19; asthma epidemic, 146; collecting, 12, 122, 145; crowdsourced, 116, 117, 149; environmental, 140, 141–48, 152, 166; patient care, 120; verification, 116; visualizations, 118, 120
datafication, 115–16, 204n19
Davis, Lily, 158, 159, 160, 177
de Certeau, Michel, 197n34
dehumidifiers, 171

diagnosis, 11, 12, 36, 40–48, 52, 53, 54, 61, 68, 71, 75, 87, 119, 123
diet, 94; vegetarian, 106
disease management, 18, 25, 83, 137–38, 182; guidelines for, 19, 134
disordered breathing, 2, 12, 16, 31, 33, 36, 37, 48, 54–55, 56, 80, 86, 87, 94, 96, 119, 121, 122, 141, 145, 180, 184, 185, 197n39; breathing techniques and, 77; chronicity of, 62; context of, 64, 75; emergence of, 35; experiencing, 102; imprint from, 83; inhalers and, 65; organizing life around, 88; problem of, 101; responding to, 57, 67, 78; seasonal variations in, 7; studies of, 10; suffering from, 85
Dorsey, Ray, 136
Dulera, taking, 69, 70
Dumit, Joseph, 64
dust, 88, 162, 167, 170, 206n17

ecology, 3, 9, 91, 185
economic dynamics, 16, 57, 89
ecosystems, 21, 162, 182
eczema, 31, 36
education: asthma and, 27; community, 150; health, 169; patient, 24, 71
EIA. See exercise-induced asthma
endotypes, 10, 38, 39
Energy Coordinating Agency, 154, 155
Englund, Harri, 74
environment, 27, 140, 160, 182; body and, 179; controlling, 78
environmental changes, 6, 51, 81, 151–52, 159, 172, 179, 206n19
environmental conditions, 7, 15, 35, 94, 118, 137–38, 143, 156, 163, 170, 179, 181; attunement to, 89; triggers from, 116
environmental control, 10, 17–18, 24, 68, 79, 80, 81–82, 170; breath

control and, 83; practicing, 82, 83, 88
environmental hazards, 36, 53, 170, 195n82
environmental health, 5, 7, 8, 18, 19, 56, 179, 194n65; dynamics of, 5; problems with, 150, 151, 175; projects, 26, 195n82
Environmental Health Perspectives (Su), 146
environmental issues, 8, 156, 172, 174, 176, 178, 179
EPA. See U.S. Environmental Protection Agency
Epstein, Steven, 201n30
ethnography, multisited, 21–28, 195n73
European Respiratory Society (ERS), 44, 62, 63, 68, 70, 198n5
exacerbations, 37, 61, 62, 63, 117, 153, 163, 198n5
exercise-induced asthma (EIA), 32, 33, 35, 41, 42, 44, 72, 74, 78, 101; described, 30–31; diagnosis of, 75
exhaling, 44, 46, 60, 76, 77, 86, 88, 96, 101, 102
exposure, 3, 10, 77, 127; atmospheric, 164; chemical, 185; environmental, 8, 57–58, 64, 116, 119, 148; prenatal, 13; reducing, 17; respiratory health, 148

FDA, 123, 147
Flovent, 72
forced vital capacity (FVC), 45
Forgetting of Air in Martin Heidegger, The (Irigary), 193n30
formaldehyde, 168
Fortun, Kim, 21, 22, 192n11
Franklin Institute, 155
Free Library of Philadelphia, 152, 153, 160

Freifeld, Clark C., 116
Frickel, Scott, 203n41

Gide, André, 111
GINA. See Global Initiative for Asthma
GlaxoSmithKline, 147
Global Initiative for Asthma (GINA), 36, 37, 38, 44, 60, 61, 62–63, 138, 198n5, 199n22, 202n39; control assessment criteria by, 126; guidelines from, 45, 126; report by, 51, 62, 67, 68
Google Play, 117, 120, 121
GPS, 115, 117–18, 136, 142, 146
Graham, Tess, 105
Grosz, Elizabeth, 196n8

Hahn, Tomie, 194n54
hay fever, 31, 32
health: climate change and, 165; issues, 154, 155, 166, 195n82; protecting, 185; responsibility for, 119; social determinants of, 20
health care, 28, 115, 169, 182; access to, 13, 15, 20, 27, 87, 182, 184; affordable, 183; ground-level, 183; providers, 24, 27, 46, 47, 52, 64, 113; responsibility for, 134; systems, 23, 119, 135, 139, 144
health insurance, 2, 27, 82, 112, 131, 135, 191n1
health management organizations (HMOs), 27, 142, 143
healthy homes, 156, 166–72, 182
Healthy Homes Program (NNCC), 151, 155, 156, 168, 169, 170
Healthy Rowhouse Project, 150
heart disease, 64
heat health emergencies, 152, 153, 155
heat islands, 162, 167
Heatline, 152, 153
heatstroke, 153

homelessness, 12, 157, 160, 161, 206n18
hospitalization, 6, 12, 13, 59, 195n77
hot spots, environmental, 145
housing, 176; affordable, 168, 185; asthma and, 150; conditions, 149, 166, 168
Housing and Community Development Act (1992), 170
humidity, 9, 162, 171
hyperresponsiveness, 37, 68
hypertension, 90, 92
hyperventilation, 77, 86, 92, 93, 94, 95, 96

Ichan School of Medicine, 137
ICS. See inhaled corticosteroids
immunoglobulin E-mediated reactions, 32
Impacts of Climate Change on Human Health in the United States: A Scientific Assessment (U.S. Global Change Research Program), 162
industrial activities, 6, 7, 192n11
inequality, 16, 20, 161, 176
inflammation, 31, 47, 62, 180
infrastructure, 8, 20, 84, 163, 175, 178, 179; chronic care, 19, 118–19, 125, 130, 131–36, 148, 181–82; environmental health design for, 185; lack of care for, 208n7; public, 176, 179
inhaled corticosteroids (ICS), 50, 51, 52, 68, 71, 72
inhalers, 14, 15, 32, 42, 66, 116, 147, 207n36; breathing and, 109–13; controller, 31, 82, 180; disordered breathing and, 65; photo of, 14; using, 75, 77, 98. See also rescue inhalers
inhaling, 60, 76, 86, 88, 95, 102; frantic, 100; normal, 101

Irigary, Luce, 193n30
iTunes Store, 126, 130

Jackson, Mark, 111, 202n38
justice: environmental, 21, 22, 150, 155, 176; social, 184

Lancet, The, 10
Landon, Matt: photo of, 21
Langstrup, Henriette, 19, 118, 119
lead, exposure to, 156, 169–70, 174
Liberty Lutheran, 154, 155
lifestyles, changes in, 10, 23, 51, 88
Live Your Life without Limits (video), 145
logbooks, 101, 102, 127
long-acting beta-2 agonists, 50
lung function, 63, 67, 133

Mankikar, Deepa, 156
Martinez, Fernando, 10, 11
Massey, Doreen, 196n8, 197n34
Massey, Laporshia: death of, 172–73, 174, 175, 207n36
Maynard, Ronald J., 78
Mayo Clinic, 121
McKeown, Patrick, 103–4, 105; photo of, 107
McPherson Library, photo of, 165
Medicaid, 14, 143
medications, 4, 5, 19, 24; adherence to, 68, 130; allergy, 14; anti-inflammatory, 31; controller, 2, 18, 53, 56, 58–59, 61, 65, 68, 71, 78, 82, 83, 87, 97, 98, 109, 110, 111–12, 143, 181; cost of, 14, 15; daily, 65, 72–73, 97–98; failure of, 8, 87, 111; prescription, 2, 3, 6, 19, 50, 64, 71, 78, 86, 87, 113, 153, 181; regimens with, 7, 23, 119; responding to, 43–44; side effects of, 64, 70, 72, 88, 110, 183; stopping, 23, 103; timescapes and, 88; using, 10,

48, 68, 69, 78, 97–98, 119, 179.
See also pharmaceuticals
medicine: Chinese, 96; complementary/
alternative, 105, 110; holistic, 93;
Tibetan, 91, 93; Western, 91, 93,
119
mental health, 15, 62, 162
Merleau-Ponty, Maurice, 196n8
Mitman, Gregg, 195n77
Mol, Annemarie, 20
mold, 3, 146, 156, 162, 167, 168, 170,
174; dangers of, 169, 171
mortality, 6, 12, 13, 14, 183, 195n77
Mount Sinai, 137, 140, 142, 146
Muñoz-Marin Elementary School,
mold outbreak at, 174
Murphy, Michelle, 194n65

NACI. See National Asthma Control
Initiative
Nading, Alex, 194n65
NAEPP. See National Asthma Educa-
tion and Prevention Program
narratives, 84, 89–94; allergy, 32;
asthma, 49; illness, 38
nasal sprays, 81
National Asthma Control Initiative
(NACI), 63, 64, 198n1, 198n14,
198n15
National Asthma Education and Pre-
vention Program (NAEPP), 44, 63,
197n32, 198n12
National Health Survey (CDC), 12
National Heart, Lung, and Blood Insti-
tute (NHLBI), 36, 38, 42, 44, 63,
198n12, 198n14
National Institute for Occupational
Safety and Health (NIOSH), 174,
207n41
National Institutes of Health, 10
National Nurse-Led Care Consortium
(NNCC), 154, 155, 156, 167, 168,
169, 170

National Science Foundation, 155
Natural Asthma Cure Workshop, 95
nebulizers, 4, 24, 51
New York Times, 13, 14, 24, 109, 112
NHLBI. See National Heart, Lung,
and Blood Institute
NIOSH. See National Institute for
Occupational Safety and Health
Nixon, Rob, 175, 176, 192n11
NNCC. See National Nurse-Led Care
Consortium
nongovernmental organizations, 22,
59, 157
Novozhilov, Andrey, 105

obesity, asthma and, 38
odors, 8
Office of Emergency Management, 152
Omalizumab, asthma treatment and,
198n41
Open Airways for Schools program,
194n67
OSIA Medical, 204n15
outcomes, 147, 182; adverse, 61, 62;
patient-reported, 137; public
health, 145; treatment, 144
overbreathing, chronic, 90, 100
Oxygen Advantage, The (McKeown),
103
ozone, 8, 152, 162, 163, 167

paint, lead in, 174
participatory epidemiology, 116
particulate matter, 167
Patient Protection and Affordable Care
Act, 131
PDPH. See Philadelphia Department of
Public Health
peak expiratory flow (PEF), 45
peak flow, measuring, 68, 118
peak flow meters, 4, 45, 46, 61, 93,
100, 132, 135, 197n32; photo of,
47; using, 47, 48

Pejham, Sam, 130
Pennsylvania Department of Environmental Protection, 152
Pennsylvania Department of Health, 149
pesticides, 3, 8, 170
pests, 3, 170, 174
pets, giving up, 81
pharmaceuticals, 7, 8, 40, 58, 59, 98, 181–82, 183, 184, 185, 202n34, 204n19; dependence on, 60, 70; development of, 12; forms of, 180; limits of, 94; success with, 111; using, 78, 82, 87, 89, 149, 202n34. *See also* medications
phenotypes, 10, 45; asthma, 32, 38–39, 55, 56, 62; classification systems for, 38, 39, 40; illustration of, 39 (fig.)
Philadelphia Corporation for Aging, Heatline of, 152
Philadelphia Department of Public Health (PDPH), 150, 151, 153, 154, 155; asthma carescape and, 165; climate and asthma working group, 166; CUSP and, 166; heat health emergencies and, 152
Philadelphia Federation of Teachers, 174; Health and Welfare Fund, 207n41
Philadelphia Health and Environment Ethnography Lab, 195n82, 205n14
Philly Healthy Schools Initiative, 174
Philly Thrive, 150
Physicians for Social Responsibility, 154
physiology, 39, 102, 179, 194n55
plants, allergenicity of, 162
political relations, 89, 171, 175, 179
pollen, 5, 6, 7, 8, 9, 23, 43, 88, 146, 167; air pollution and, 4; climate change and, 163; concentration of, 162–63; counts, 143; pollution and, 164; weather conditions and, 164
pollution, 9, 43, 94, 153; density, 162; indoor/outdoor, 167–68; industrial, 7; pollen and, 164
polycyclic aromatic hydrocarbons, 8
poverty, 14, 15, 26, 149, 166, 175, 206n19; asthma and, 150, 173, 174, 207n38; legacy of, 179; living in, 12, 171
prevalence rates, 3, 12, 144, 163, 195n77, 205n2; African Americans and, 13; childhood, 149; climate change and, 185; Hispanics and, 13; racial disparities in, 13, 15; whites and, 13; women and, 13, 15
prevention, 2, 5, 10, 14, 15, 17, 30, 36, 68, 72, 145, 164, 180, 183; emphasis on, 181
Propeller Health, 116, 117, 130, 137, 142, 144–45, 148, 182; asthma care and, 147; mobile asthma app and, 26, 115, 141, 146; success for, 204n34
Proust, Marcel, 111, 202n38
public health, 17, 22, 38, 63, 64, 78, 140, 145, 146, 153, 176, 179, 182; agencies, 164; expenditures, 143; interventions, 149; literature, 175; organizations, 36; records, 136; services, 117, 121; studies, 130
Public Health Institute, 165, 166, 206n25
Puig de la Bellacasa, María, 18, 89, 192n17, 194n60, 200n10
Pulmonary-Allergy Drugs Advisory Committee, 10
pulmonary function, 34, 44, 46, 48, 92
pulmonary performance, 20, 37, 46; tests, 8, 45, 93

race, 12, 22
racism: environmental, 149, 161; structural, 175, 179
Rackemann, Francis, 196–97n25
radon, 170
ragweed, 162
Ramirez, Maria: photo of, 165
Regional Asthma Management Program, 194n67
relations: human–nonhuman, 6, 8, 28, 203n3; social, 158; strain on, 54
relaxation, 76–77, 102; breathing and, 94–99
Renesselear Polytechnic Institute (RPI), 22, 23, 80
Reno, Joshua, 74
rescue inhalers, 1–2, 48, 58, 65, 66, 68, 97, 111, 117, 142, 181; access to, 183; GPS sensors on, 26; photo of, 14; thunderstorm asthma and, 5; using, 2–3, 10, 52, 73, 76, 145, 177, 180
research, 40, 41, 78, 83, 91, 115, 136, 145, 159, 183; archive of, 103; BBT, 105; crowdsourced data for, 116; interdisciplinary, 21; medical, 79, 105; public health, 121, 146, 151; treatment, 113
ResearchKit, 136, 137, 138, 141
respiration, 73, 93, 106; habits of, 102; rates, 90, 99, 107, 201n24
respiratory disease, understanding/controlling, 116
respiratory infections, 168, 169
respiratory rates, 90, 99, 107, 201n24
responsibility, 63, 64, 80, 97, 125, 127, 134, 167, 185; civic, 79; individual/collective, 8, 161–62; personal, 97, 119, 126, 143
rhythms, 18, 88, 98, 106, 109, 181; breathing, 89, 90; narrative, 89–94; respiratory, 57, 93, 99, 179; therapeutic, 192n17

risk factors, 13, 62, 117
River Wards, 150, 153, 167, 168, 175, 206n17
Roberto Clemente Middle School, mold outbreak at, 174
Roseman, Jerry, 207n41

SABA. See short-acting beta-2 adrenergic agonist
Salbutamol, 1
School District of Philadelphia, 150, 172, 174, 207n36
seasonal variations, 6, 7, 9, 18, 23
self-care, 127, 140
Self Care Movement, 127
SEPTA. See Southeastern Pennsylvania Transportation Authority
short-acting beta-2 adrenergic agonist (SABA), 30, 50
side effects, 63, 71, 98; medication, 64, 70, 72, 88, 110, 183
sleep disorders, 86, 200n3
sleeping positions, 106
Slow Violence and the Environmentalism of the Poor (Nixon), 175
smartphones, 25, 131, 136, 142, 146
smoke, 8, 44, 162
social circumstances, 7, 78, 89
socioeconomic conditions, 15, 84, 163
Southeastern Pennsylvania Transportation Authority (SEPTA), 177, 178, 179
spirometers, 45, 46, 61, 93, 133, 197n32
spraygrounds, 152
Stalmatski, Alexander, 96, 105, 107–8
Stark, Jennifer, 105
Stark, Russell, 105
"Staying Cool in a Changing Climate" (workshop), 152, 154, 156, 158; photo of, 154, 165
steroids, 58, 70, 110
Stewart, Kathleen, 36, 193n53

Stop Asthma Naturally (Byrne-Ralfs and McKeown), display for, 104 (fig.)

strep throat, 71

stress, 8, 98, 99, 101; BBT and, 96; psychosomatic, 49

Su, Jason G., 146

symptoms, 9, 11, 23, 37, 40–41, 43, 52, 53, 55, 72, 97, 100, 140, 177; air quality and, 51; allergy, 112; asthma, 2, 3, 6, 17, 34, 112; BBT and, 181; decline of, 99; EIA, 74–75; managing, 67, 80, 118; medical care for, 4; nighttime, 126; poor control of, 62; preventing, 2; respiratory, 44, 62, 153, 167; responding to, 17; seasonal, 81; self-reported, 38; triggering, 116, 141, 162

teaching tools, BBE, 95 (fig.)

technology, 19, 123, 135, 147, 183; biomedical, 25, 79; chemical, 6; digital, 6; environmental, 203n3; normalization, 78; personal, 117, 125, 130, 136; self-care, 100; studies, 16, 179

technoscientific elements, 7, 16, 19

temperatures, 7, 162, 163, 167

temporality, 11, 19, 52, 60, 158, 194n60

Thrift, Nigel: geography and, 193n53

Th2-inflammation hypothesis, 11, 192n27

timescales, 89, 91, 94, 182

timescapes, 18, 32, 89, 91, 94, 102, 161, 178, 179; ecological, 19; environmental, 84; medications and, 88

Tracy, Greg, 147

Training Institute of Buteyko Educators, 105

transportation, 20, 176, 177; public, 161, 178, 185

treatment, 5, 12, 18, 52, 80, 113, 123, 198n41, 199n22; alternative, 78; controller, 44; discussion of, 200n1; drug, 55–56; nonpharmaceutical, 60, 70, 98; resistance to, 202n39; trends in, 24

triggers, 3, 9, 9 (fig.), 33, 50, 54, 55, 56, 70, 72, 88, 101, 141, 167, 199n38; asthma, 127, 170; behavioral, 52; buildup of, 168; changing atmosphere of, 158–66; controlling, 82; eliminating/avoiding, 81, 83; environmental, 46, 52, 73, 116, 117; potential, 17; user-reported, 137

Trnka, Susanna: work of, 195n83

United Mountain Defense, 21

University of Pittsburgh Asthma Institute, 38

U.S. Department of Housing and Urban Development, 156

U.S. Environmental Protection Agency (EPA), 140, 205n12; AQI of, 152–53, 169, 207n30

U.S. Food and Drug Administration, 10, 125

USGCRP. *See* U.S. Global Change Research Program

U.S. Global Change Research Program (USGCRP), 162, 163, 164, 167, 168, 175, 207n26

U.S. National Institutes of Health, 36

USSR Cabinet of Ministers Committee for Science and Technology, 92

Van Sickle, David, 26, 117, 146

vehicle idling, laws against, 15

ventilation, 93, 166, 167, 168, 170

Ventolin, 42

viruses, 7, 8, 42, 44, 48, 51, 52, 65, 70, 127

volatile organic compounds, 168
Voyage app, The, 135

water damage, 168, 174
W. C. Bryant Promise Academy, 172,
    173, 174
weather, 44, 143, 159, 160, 164, 165;
    extreme, 167; patterns, 3, 163
Wenzel, Sally, 38, 40
West Philadelphia Senior Community
    Center, 153, 158
wheezing, 1, 2, 8, 11, 24, 30, 35, 36,
    37, 41, 44, 52, 58, 65, 66, 69, 75

Whitmarsh, Ian: work of, 195n83
Wiebe, David: BBT and, 110
Wilson, Dr., 123, 124, 143–44
Wolf-Meyer, Matthew, 192n17, 200n3
workshops, 157, 165, 168, 171, 172,
    182; BBT, 86, 87, 88, 95, 96
World Health Organization, 36

Yakovic-Fredericksen, Sasha, 105
Yakovic-Fredericksen, Thomas, 105

Zerbo, Russ, 152, 156, 159; photo of,
    154

A L I S O N   K E N N E R is assistant professor in the Department of Politics and the Center for Science, Technology, and Society at Drexel University, where she is also involved with the Institute for Energy and Environment in the College of Engineering and the Urban Health Collaborative in the Dornsife School of Public Health.